praise for Tracey Mallett's

SUPER FIT MAMA

"*Super Fit Mama* takes all the guesswork and guilt out of maintaining fitness during pregnancy and in the weeks after delivery. Tracey's detailed workouts along with pictures to demonstrate will have you feeling like Madonna with your own personal trainer!"

> —Victoria McEvoy, MD, Assistant in Pediatrics at Harvard Medical School and Medical Director and Chief of Pediatrics at Mass General West Medical Group

"Tracey Mallett offers all the fitness and nutrition information you need throughout your pregnancy and beyond. The workouts are challenging and fun; the recipes are delicious, nutritious and easy to make. *Super Fit Mama* is the must-have companion book for every Mom."

> —Mary Jane Horton, *Plum* Magazine Editor-in-Chief

"*Super Fit Mama* really delivers the motivation! It's fun, fresh, and feels like Tracey is a friend, who knows what it's like juggling the 24/7 demands of work, family and trying to stay fit and healthy. I especially love her lists of helpful hints for each trimester! This book is has something for everyone, no matter where they're at in pregnancy or after delivery. The exercises are easy to do and better yet, they really work."

> —Barbara Dehn, RN, MS, NP, Women's Health Nurse Practitioner

"*Super Fit Mama* is the essential guide for eating healthy and staying fit during pregnancy and for getting your body back quickly and safely after delivery. Tracey Mallett has done an outstanding job putting together a program that's not only medically sound, but doable and realistic enough for even a busy new mom to follow!"

> —Andrew Larson, MD, FACS, author of *The Gold Coast Cure* series and *The Whole Foods Diet Cookbook*

"I know that as a working woman it's hard to fit exercise into your daily routine and when you're pregnant you can feel simply exhausted. But Tracey's practical instruction teaches you how to work in fitness in small increments of time. This is a 'must-read!'"

> —Alison Rhodes, "The Safety Mom," Founder, Safety Mom Enterprises

"We are so tired after having a baby, but after reading *Super Fit Mama*, I became inspired. Tracey's style is uplifting and contagious. A new mommy will want to eat better and look hot after reading this book!"

—Kimberley Clayton Blaine, MA, MFT, founder of www.TheGoToMom.TV, author of *Mommy Confidence*

"Informative and inspiring, *Super Fit Mama* should be required reading for every pregnant (and post-partum) woman determined to get her former body back. Motherhood is a marathon—and if you follow Tracey's lead, you'll hit the starting line in the best shape of your life."

—Jenna McCarthy, author of *The Parent Trip: From High Heels and Parties to Highchairs and Potties*

"Simply put, *Super Fit Mama* is a must-have for all mothers-to-be. Dealing with a topic so full of myths and misconceptions, Tracey expertly blends science with real world examples, finally bringing exercise and pregnancy into the 21st century."

—Tom Holland, MS, CSCS, Exercise Physiologist

"Having a baby changes everything . . . but your body does not have to be unrecognizable forever! Tracey Mallett skillfully empowers expectant and new mothers with the tools to reclaim your bodies, refresh your minds after sleepless nights, and look better than ever!"

—Vonda Wright, MD, Orthopedic Surgeon, new mother at 40, and author of *Fitness After 40: How to Stay Strong at Any Age*

"Indispensable for anyone looking to stay fit during and after pregnancy. Tracey's fitness plan is brilliantly laid out by trimester so a pregnant woman never needs to wonder what is or isn't safe (bonus points for detailing foods and workouts that actually help keep first trimester nausea at bay). She also provides everything from simple recipes to easy workouts for moms on the go, saving them what they need the most during those first few months after baby's arrival—time!"

—Kate Ward, Editor, TheBump.com

SUPER FIT MAMA

SUPER
FIT
MAMA

**STAY FIT DURING PREGNANCY AND
GET YOUR BODY BACK AFTER BABY**

TRACEY MALLETT

Da Capo
∞
LIFE
LONG

A Member of the Perseus Books Group

DESIGN BY JANE RAESE
Set in 12-point Bulmer

Cataloging-in-Publication data for this book is available from the Library of Congress.

First Da Capo Press edition 2009
ISBN: 978-1-60094-031-6

Published by Da Capo Press
A Member of the Perseus Books Group
www.dacapopress.com

Da Capo Press books are available at special discounts for bulk purchases in the U.S. by corporations, institutions, and other organizations. For more information, please contact the Special Markets Department at the Perseus Books Group, 2300 Chestnut Street, Suite 200, Philadelphia, PA, 19103, or call (800) 810-4145, ext. 5000, or e-mail special.markets@perseusbooks.com.

10 9 8 7 6 5 4 3 2

Dedicated to my Mom, Nan, and my beautiful children Amber and Ty
for helping me be the best possible Mom I can be.

CONTENTS

Merrill Sue Lewen, MD

When I met Tracey Mallett in 2001, she was pregnant with her first child. I had just moved to Southern California and had joined the same practice as her OB/GYN. Tracey and I instantly bonded over our common interest in exercise and pregnancy, and two years later I delivered her second child.

During both of my pregnancies, I had exercised to the bitter end, and I had always found that the women in my practice who exercised during pregnancy felt better about themselves and being pregnant than those who didn't. At the time, this was becoming Tracey's forte. I began sending pregnant and postpartum patients to her practice, and later, my gynecology patients benefited from her studio's physical therapists. Tracey was able to tap into the individual patients' needs. Her knowledge of this field never ceases to amaze me.

Exercise has become a modern American obsession. Luckily, it is one of our few healthy obsessions. In a world where being thin is so highly regarded, being pregnant can present a challenge for women. Giving up one's regular workout routine and watching the scale go up and up can drive some women to the depths of depression at what should be one of the most exciting and wonderful times of their lives. Our generation knows not to smoke or drink during pregnancy and not to take certain medications and supplements. We know what foods to avoid, and most of us have considered whether we want to choose organic. But most pregnant women are not well educated about how to exercise safely during pregnancy. One's current regimen may be just fine (yes, your heart rate can go above 140!), or it may not be (you could fall off that mountain bike pretty hard!). But answers to the questions women have about exercise during pregnancy are not always intuitive.

In *Super Fit Mama*, Tracey has brilliantly compiled medically sound facts regarding pregnancy and fitness. She caters to the pregnant woman of today who has that healthy obsession for staying fit, reminding her that the demands on her body while pregnant are significant, and that first and foremost she must *listen to that body!*

There are as many answers to the question of how to stay in shape while pregnant as there are variations of a latte at Starbucks, and Tracey has put these together in a practical, entertaining, and personal way. She dispels myths about exercise during pregnancy, describes how to exercise safely in each trimester while enjoying your changing pregnant body, explains how to handle exercise in the postpartum period, and provides invaluable nutritional tips. Remember, after your pregnancy your body will take time to get back to normal. Your body will be larger than it was before your pregnancy for at least a year. This is not always an easy thing to accept. But if you follow Tracey's program, you will soon be a "Super Fit Mama."

Tracy's regimen also helps those who are overly concerned about their weight to recognize that when it comes to exercise, more is not necessarily better. Her great website (www.TraceyMallett.com) is another resource for these type A pregnant women, a place where they can go for close to constant support regarding these issues.

Tracey has managed the difficult task of rolling all of these issues into one, combining her understanding of how a woman feels while pregnant and postpartum with a practical, safe, but serious exercise regimen. Being pregnant is often a vulnerable time for women, and it is extremely important to know where to turn for good information that is truly helpful. *Super Fit Mama* empowers women with Tracey acting as a guide, helping them achieve their goals with a program that is both effective and highly motivating.

As a woman grows with a pregnancy, and then as her family grows postpartum, it is easy for her to become overwhelmed by the awesome but sometimes uncomfortable changes taking place in her body as well as the more complex ones taking place in her life. Having the support and excellent information that Tracey provides in *Super Fit Mama* will help you enjoy these changes as you move through this very challenging and wonderful time in life.

Merrill Sue Lewen, MD, is in private practice at Town and Country Gynecology in Houston, Texas.

Howard S. Kaufman, MD

In *Super Fit Mama*, international fitness expert Tracey Mallett presents essential information for new mothers in a comprehensive plan that promotes long-term health and wellness through healthy diet and exercise. In addition, Tracey continues her mission to tackle critical women's health issues that have previously been considered taboo. One such issue is pelvic floor disorders. Tracey's program stresses the importance of health, exercise, diet, and lifestyle during pregnancy and after delivery, which are some of the most critical times for the development of these problems. *Super Fit Mama* can help women prevent or remedy these debilitating conditions.

Many new mothers aren't familiar with the problems that can be associated with delivering a baby, but the statistics of pelvic floor disorders are staggering. By age fifty-five, more than half of women suffer one or more of the problems caused by pelvic floor dysfunction; by age seventy-five, this increases to three-fourths of women. One of these problems is urinary incontinence, a problem affecting more than 20 million women in the United States. In addition to childbirth, obesity and aging also contribute to our national epidemic of pelvic floor disorders. These conditions include bowel and bladder dysfunction like urinary incontinence, overactive bladder, and loss of bowel control, all of which can lead to sexual dysfunction and a number of psychosocial and emotional disturbances, ranging from anxiety to social isolation and exclusion.

Many women who seek treatment at our Center for Pelvic Floor Disorders at the Keck School of Medicine of the University of Southern California have been told that these conditions are "part of aging," "natural for women who have had children," or "something that you'll have to live with." While these statements may reflect the current thought paradigm among many health-care providers, fortunately they are simply not true.

The current state-of-the-art care for prevention and treatment of pelvic floor disorders starts with pelvic floor muscle exercises. These exercises have been proven to reduce the incidence of urinary incontinence during pregnancy and after delivery and are safe and effective in treating incontinence in women decades after childbirth. Pelvic floor muscle exercises and core conditioning are also known to improve many aspects of sexual function and can increase sexual desire, satisfaction, performance, and achievement of orgasm.

Super Fit Mama includes many of the important exercises that can help women prevent or treat these disorders. As a result, women who follow Tracey's comprehensive plan should benefit from improved long-term strength and quality of life, which may decrease their need for invasive surgical procedures in the future.

> *Howard S. Kaufman, MD, is associate*
> *professor of clinical surgery and*
> *obstetrics and gynecology and director of*
> *the Center for Pelvic Floor Disorders at*
> *Keck School of Medicine at the*
> *University of Southern California.*

CHAPTER 1

IT'S TIME TO BE A SUPER FIT MAMA!

ONGRATULATIONS! YOU'RE ABOUT TO BEGIN THE WONDER-ful journey of pregnancy and parenthood. Regardless of where you are along this adventure—just starting it, somewhere in the middle, or postpartum—*Super Fit Mama* is for you.

Imagine, just days, weeks, or months ago you saw two lines on your pregnancy test or heard your doctor say, "You're pregnant," and suddenly your whole world has changed. Though my children are now ages six and four, I remember those days like they were yesterday. After peeing on a few boxes full of sticks, I was thrilled to find out I was pregnant and about to become a mother. But I do admit that I was also scared. Scared to watch my very fit body transform into, well, into I don't know what. Would I be one of those petite people with just a basketball belly, I wondered, or would I have one of those bodies that seemed to blow up in every single direction imaginable? (After adding 55 pounds to my five-foot, three-inch frame, I turned out to be the latter.)

In order to explain why I wrote *Super Fit Mama*, let me share a little bit of my journey from pregnancy to motherhood. It's a journey I've taken twice, and I've learned some great lessons along the way. When I was pregnant with my first child, Amber, I started out worrying how I'd handle the inevitable weight gain. After all, as a fitness expert, I'm in an industry where people are not forgiving if you have a few bulges hanging over your yoga pants even if you ARE pregnant. But I decided right from the beginning that I'd enjoy this pregnancy to its fullest. And boy, did I enjoy it: curly fries, creamed mashed potatoes (my biggest craving), and just a little too much dessert. I remember thinking, "I'm plumping up anyway, so what's a few extra calories going to do to my butt?" I repeatedly told myself, "I'm eating for two!" (Sound familiar?) But I admit, it wasn't all fun and French fries. Some days I'd stare at my expanding waistline and wonder if I'd kissed my abs good-bye forever or if I'd ever fit into my favorite pair of jeans again. Eventually I did come to my healthy senses and face facts: The extra 300 calories a day that you're supposed to eat through your pregnancy for the healthy development of the baby should not consist of nutritionally empty cookies.

During this first pregnancy, I decided to shoot my *3 in 1 Pregnancy System* fitness DVD. After all, I'd been a personal trainer for many years and, despite a few pregnancy pig-outs, I knew how important it was to keep your body healthy and strong by exercising during each trimester. Yet once I delivered Amber, I didn't have the confidence with my new Mommy body to release the DVD into the world. I really thought the weight would easily slip off once my little one was born, but unfortunately most of it was staying put. That realization was devastating. For some reason I thought being a personal trainer and someone who had been exercising her whole life would give me some sort of "get out of your maternity clothes free pass." I thought I'd come home from the hospital and in a few weeks or so would be wearing my regular jeans. I have to say, it was a horrible moment when I reached for those pants and realized I couldn't even get them up past my thighs.

After a few weeks of this frustration, I had totally lost confidence in myself and my ability to achieve my goals. How could I act like an authority on fitness when I couldn't even whip my own postpartum body into shape? I certainly didn't know whose body I was looking at in the mirror. Like so many women in this position, I was so overwhelmed with motherhood.

Then one day I was standing in front of the mirror trying on bathing suits for the first time post-baby. I looked at my bulging, shapeless body and thought, "Oh it's not so bad. I'm a Mom now, this is how my body is supposed to look." But as soon as this thought went through my head, I knew that it was time to take action! I decided that "being a mom" was no excuse for feeling uncomfortable in my own skin. I knew that I needed to create a plan for myself to slim down and get in shape that fit into my life as a mother. Gone were the days where I had long stretches of time to exercise and the endless energy to do so. I needed an effective, efficient plan that I could easily squeeze into my hectic and often unpredictable life with a baby.

As a result, I created "Sexy in 6," the fitness and eating program that eventually became the basis of my first book. The goal was to break exercise down into small, manageable chunks that fit into the real life of moms the world over (real moms, not the celebrity variety who have nannies, trainers, and cooks at their beck and call). At the same time, I used the Sexy in 6 plan with an array of my personal training clients, and when they reaped fabulous results and shared it with their friends, I knew it was time to formally put it together into a book for women everywhere. The result, *Sexy in 6: Sculpt Your Body with the 6 Minute Quick-Blast Workout,* came out in January 2008. I am so proud of it and of all the women who have written in and told me how it's changed their life.

However, I've also received a flood of letters from moms-to-be asking me if it's okay to use the Sexy in 6 program while pregnant or immediately postpartum. For the most part, it is okay, but I knew they could reap better results with a more targeted, structured program that specifically addressed the diet and exercise needs of pregnant women and new moms. The result is Super Fit Mama, a healthy exercise and eating plan that can help you stay in shape and feel fantastic while you're pregnant and then get your pre-baby body back fast once your bundle of joy arrives.

To make sure that the Super Fit Mama program would give women the world over terrific results, I recruited a group of forty-five women to give it a test drive. I call these awesome moms "Team Mallett."

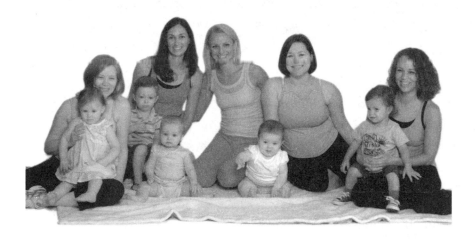

The tricky part was this: Most of the women on Team Mallett were pregnant with their second child and the rest worked full time. My challenge was creating a workout that would fit into their busy lives, and, phew, I'm happy to say it did. The women loved that the workouts could be broken into small chunks that they could squeeze into their unpredictable schedules. I was so proud when they collectively lost over 700 pounds! I was so inspired by so many of their stories, and I hope you will be, too.

In *Super Fit Mama*, you'll find workouts that are ideal for both pregnancy and postpartum. The workouts are short, manageable chunks of exercise that have been specifically designed to recruit as many muscles at one time as possible to achieve the most efficient workout. Ideally, you can use this book starting in pregnancy, but if you pick it up postpartum, that's fine, too (the pregnancy section will always come in handy for next time around!). You will also find a food plan, nutrition tips, and recipes that will satisfy any craving and get you into your favorite jeans fast. And because all the workouts are designed for moms, they can all be done at home with very little equipment. In fact, all you'll need is two sets of dumbbells (3 and 5 pounds if you're new to fitness or just returning to exercise, and 5 to 8 pounds for the more experienced exerciser), a mat, and supportive sneakers (make sure you get running shoes if you plan to run for your cardio, since these provide the most cushioning).

I truly believe that all women deserve to feel fit, strong, sexy, and confident, and that is the goal of *Super Fit Mama.* It's a plan that you can easily fit into your life, and it's flexible enough to keep you interested and excited about living a healthy lifestyle—during pregnancy, immediately afterward, and beyond. So slip on your workout clothes and get ready to feel like a Super Fit Mama from this day forward!

Team Mallett Success Story

* *

Marley Majcher, a.k.a. "The Party Goddess," 38, Pasadena, CA

Lost

30 pounds

3 dress sizes

23 total inches

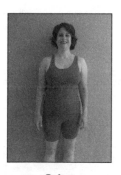
Before

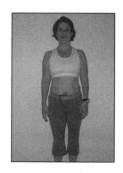
After

• • • • •

After having her third child, Marley was "totally depressed" about the way she looked. "I know you're not going to look model-ready two days after you have a baby, but I still felt bummed out," she says. "The only thing that made me feel like I was getting back into the swing of things was being proactive." As soon as her doctor gave her the okay to exercise, Marley began exercising to my DVDs and doing the Super Fit Mama program. "Not only did I have more energy, I finally felt empowered and like I was actually molding my flab into something a little more sculpted and desirable," Marley says.

What she loved most about the Super Fit Mama workouts was that she didn't need a gym membership and could do them with little equipment. "I love that the exercises are quick and easy to do anywhere—from the living room to a hotel room," she says.

Marley realized that exercising and eating right do more than get you into your skinny jeans. "My old mentality was to think about how many sweets I could eat and still lose weight," she says. "But, through the Super Fit Mama plan, I realized that I had to switch to thinking about the big picture and how I want to be healthy, not just slim." This has helped her take a "no more excuses" view of getting in shape. Marley is not only a mother of three, but a super Mompreneur with little to no time of her own. "Now that I've dropped 30+ pounds (and counting!) I can truly see the light at the end of the tunnel," she says. "And I'm on fire in all aspects of my life!"

CHAPTER 2

FIRST TRIMESTER FITNESS
On Your Mark, Get Set, Go!

THE AMERICAN COLLEGE OF OBSTETRICIANS AND GYNECOLO-gists recommends a weight gain during pregnancy of 25–35 pounds if you start out at a normal body weight. (You should gain 28–40 pounds if you're underweight and 15–25 if you're over-weight.) As I mentioned earlier, I put on a whopping 55 pounds during my first pregnancy because I convinced myself that I was eating for two and that I was *supposed* to be plumping up. It was quite hard to lose all that weight afterward. When I got pregnant the second time, I wanted to make that pregnancy better and healthier, something that also helped me slim down faster when my second child was born.

YOUR BABY

- By 4 weeks your baby is about the size of a poppy seed.
- By 8 weeks your baby is about the size of a kidney bean.
- By 10 weeks your baby is about the size of a kumquat.
- By 12 weeks your baby is about the size of a lime.

Clearly, I'm not the only woman who has gained way too much weight during pregnancy. In fact, one in four expectant mothers puts on 40 pounds or more, according to the Institute of Medicine. What's amazing to me is that most of the literature at the doctor's office or in books tells you what foods to avoid. However, there's not a whole lot of guidance as far as what foods to *eat*. But don't worry, *Super Fit Mama* will give you the essential information on nutrition to keep you on a healthy track so that your post-pregnancy body isn't one that's forever covered in baby fat!

EXERCISE IN THE FIRST TRIMESTER

Light to moderate exercise is an important part of feeling your best during pregnancy and bouncing back into shape afterward. Working out gives you energy and, according to the American College of Obstetricians and Gynecologists (ACOG), may provide some relief from pregnancy symptoms such as backaches, constipation, and bloating and swelling as well as reduce your risk of gestational diabetes and help you sleep better (something that's not easy, especially as your belly expands and your baby starts kickboxing). For some women, like me, exercise also helps curb morning sickness. Experts also say that breaking a sweat while pregnant may help soothe the pain of labor and that it can help you maintain a positive outlook about yourself, your pregnancy, and labor and delivery.

During the first trimester, I recommend that you follow the same exercise plan that I have outlined for what I call "Body After Baby Phase I." You will be returning to these exercises in weeks 7–19 postpartum, and they are described in detail in Chapter 7. If you begin to feel uncomfortable with these, move on to the exercises presented in Chapter 3 for the second-trimester plan. Later in this chapter I provide small pictures of the Chapter 7 exercises for your reference. You can also do some extra cardio exercises such as walking or swimming, following the guidelines provided below.

Keep your skin in tip-top shape during pregnancy and you just may ward off those dreaded stretch marks. Though experts say genetics plays a role in whether or not you get them, I say do all you can to prevent them. My favorite way is with Mama Mio Tummy Rub Butter, a hydrating cream that contains omega 3, 6, and 9 fatty acids, and was a reported favorite of celebs like Christina Aguilera and Jessica Alba when they were pregnant. Look for all their products at www.mamamio.com.

Of course, before resuming exercise or starting any new program, *always ask your physician or midwife if it's safe for you to work out.* And even when you've been given the green light, make sure that you really listen to your body's cues, because it will tell you when you're tired or if you're overexerting yourself.

COMMON PHYSICAL CHANGES IN THE FIRST TRIMESTER

- You should gain about 3 to 5 pounds during this trimester, and often the first place that plumps up is your breasts.
- Your uterus will begin to grow in size in order to house your baby. As a result you may feel little twinges of pain on either side of your belly called "round ligament pain."
- Your bladder will be compressed thanks to that growing uterus, so you may find yourself having to pee more often.
- You may be constipated (something an estimated 20 to 50 percent of pregnant women experience). The hormone progesterone causes the muscles in the wall of the bowel to relax, so they're not making the contractions needed to help move things along. If constipation persists, it's advised to consult with your doctor; it could be that there's too much iron in your prenatal vitamins.
- You may be really (and quite embarrassingly) gassy! Again, the slowing down of your digestive tract means that your stomach is full longer than usual. That and the resulting constipation can cause gassiness. Also, pregnancy itself may not be the culprit, but certain things you're doing as a result of the pregnancy, such as eating more calcium, fruits, veggies, and other fiber-rich foods.
- You may experience acid reflux—a burning sensation around your chest often called heartburn (though it has nothing to do with your heart). An old wives' tale claims that heartburn means that your baby will be born with a full head of hair, but your baby's locks aren't the problem. High levels of progesterone cause the muscle that sits between the esophagus and stomach to relax, and when this happens, acids from your stomach can move upward more easily. And as your uterus grows, the pressure it puts on your stomach may also push these acids up.

During the first trimester your body is working overtime to form the baby's tiny organs, skeleton, and nervous system, and you may find yourself very tired and experiencing nausea from the hormonal surge. If so, work out at a lower intensity or take time off. Remember, pregnancy is not the time to dramatically increase your fitness level. According to the American College of Sports Medicine, your exercise intensity during pregnancy shouldn't exceed your pre-pregnancy levels.

Cardio Exercise During Pregnancy

Did you know that when you're pregnant, your blood volume increases by 50 percent? This facilitates the exchange of respiratory gases, nutrients, and metabolites between you and your baby and also serves to reduce the impact of maternal blood loss at delivery. As a result of all this extra blood circulating in your body, your heart rate is higher (even at rest), especially in the first trimester. The additional blood volume also causes you to take deeper, faster breaths and lowers your blood pressure.

Cardiovascular exercise during pregnancy is a great way to build endurance, improve blood circulation, and strengthen your muscles (not to mention that it helps alleviate that oh-so-annoying pregnancy-induced

IMPORTANT EXERCISE GUIDELINES

Though doing at least 30 minutes of moderate exercise per day during pregnancy is encouraged (unlike in your Grandma's days when women were pretty much told not to move for nine months), there are some guidelines that you should follow, according to the American College of Obstetricians and Gynecologists (ACOG):

- If you've previously been exercising and have the green light from your MD or midwife, you may continue your exercise program.
- If you're completely new to exercise, consult with your MD or midwife before starting any new exercise plan.
- Don't exercise at all if you have heart or lung disease, incompetent cervix or cerclage, placenta previa, ruptured membranes, or preeclampsia or are carrying multiples and thus have a risk of premature labor.
- Regulating your body temperature is really important. To make sure you keep cool, drink enough water before, during, and after exercise; wear loose-fitting clothes that wick sweat away from the body; and avoid exercising in high heat. This also means skipping hot yoga (a.k.a. Bikram Yoga), which is done in a room heated at around 90–100°F.
- Never exercise to complete exhaustion.
- Avoid lying on your back during the second and third trimesters.
- Avoid activities that up your risk of falling or having abdominal trauma, such as basketball, soccer, in-line skating, downhill skiing, horseback riding, ice hockey, gymnastics, and racquet sports like racquetball and squash.
- Save scuba diving for a postpartum vacation, since it's not safe at *any time* while pregnant.
- Avoid activities at altitudes higher than 6,000 feet.
- During these nine months, stop exercising IMMEDIATELY and call your doctor as soon as possible if you experience vaginal bleeding, muscle weakness, calf pain or swelling, dizziness, headache, overheating, pain in the pubic bone area, shortness of breath, cramps, chest pain, severe nausea, or leakage of amniotic fluid.

constipation). It also helps sustain increased blood flow to the skin, which helps to cool your body. However, it's important to stay well hydrated, prevent overheating, and refrain from taking part in any activity that may cause abdominal trauma.

According to ACOG, you can safely engage in 30 minutes or more of moderate exercise on most, if not all, days of the week. Walking, swimming, riding a stationary bike, using the elliptical, and doing low-impact aerobics are perfect cardio options as your pregnancy progresses, since these activities don't put any pressure on your joints, loose ligaments, or pelvic floor. However, if you were jogging or spinning prior to your pregnancy, then it's probably safe to continue.

If you're new to doing cardio, start off easily by walking at a slow to moderate pace. Then, as you feel stronger and move into the second trimester, you can bump up the intensity a little. Cross-training is the best option, especially through pregnancy when your body is going through so many physiological changes, because it will ensure that you're not overusing certain muscles. Working a wide range of muscles can help you steer clear of injury and keep you moving as normally as possible over the next nine months. Of course, you also don't want to overdo exercising when you're pregnant because extreme fatigue, injury, and excess stress on your body from *too much* exercise can prevent the baby from getting enough nutrients and oxygen.

Finding the Right Intensity

The intensity of exercise during pregnancy matters. The more intense your workout, the more blood flow and oxygen going toward your muscles and away from your growing baby. But how do you find a level that is intense enough to be beneficial, but also safe enough that you can be sure you are not depriving your baby of anything he or she needs?

Up until recently, pregnant women were told to monitor their intensity by keeping their heart rates no higher than 140 beats per minute (bpm),

CARDIO NO NO'S

Don't do these exercises while pregnant:

1. Fast interval training
2. Plyometrics (jumping, hopping, etc.)
3. Fast-paced aerobics, or pumping your hands over your head for a long period of time
4. Impact kickboxing, which can cause trauma to your belly (nonimpact cardio kickboxing is okay as long as you feel comfortable; however, as your pregnancy progresses balance will become an issue)

and this advice is still often repeated in women's magazines, other information guides, and even by some doctors and midwives. However, many experts believe that this rule of thumb may not apply to people who were regular exercisers before pregnancy. A woman's age may also make a difference. As a result, it seems that a potentially better way to determine intensity is to use "rate of perceived exertion" (RPE) instead of target heart rates.

RPE is simply the level of intensity that you feel you are experiencing. It is somewhat subjective, but that doesn't mean you have nothing to base it on. How hard are you breathing? How fast is your heart beating? Are you sweating? Can you carry on a conversation? Are you comfortable, or are you starting to feel tired? There are different RPE scales used, but in the Super Fit Mama program I decided to use a simple scale of 1 to 10, with 1 being no exertion at all and 10 being maximal (see the RPE chart in Chapter 7). Throughout your entire pregnancy, use the RPE scale to gauge how hard you're working out, and make sure your intensity is no more than a 7–8 on the chart. Another simple way to monitor yourself is the talk test. You should always be able to carry on a conversation while you work out, and if you can't, you're working out too intensely.

Finally, remember that your heart rate will be much higher than it was before you became pregnant. It may take as long as 15 minutes for your heart to recover to resting rate following a workout, so the cooldown is a critical part of your workout. The bottom line here and throughout this book is to listen to your body. Stop exercising when you feel fatigued, and never, ever exercise to exhaustion.

Exercising Your Abs

Before we go any further, we need to have a quick but important abdominal and pelvic floor anatomy lesson. Understanding how your abs function and their purpose through pregnancy and beyond will help prevent injuries, give you the knowledge you need to achieve a strong core, and help your stretched-out abs recover more quickly post-pregnancy.

There are four layers of abdominal muscle. The transverse abdominals (the deepest layer), the internal and external obliques (the waist), and the rectus abdominus (which is responsible for those enviable six-pack muscles). Beginning in the second trimester, the pressure of the expanding uterus on the rectus abdominus can force these muscles to separate. This condition is called *diastasis recti*. Regularly check to see if you have this separation using the assessment tool in Chapter 3 so that you don't perform

Diagram of the abdominals

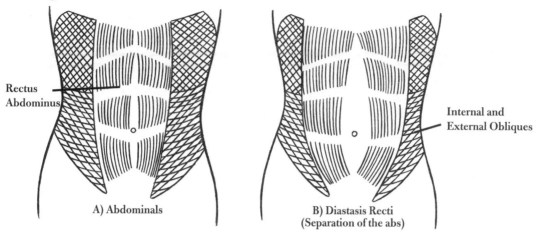

Rectus Abdominus

Internal and External Obliques

A) Abdominals

B) Diastasis Recti (Separation of the abs)

movements that will make the gap larger. In this book, exercises that are safe to perform with a diastasis through the second and third trimesters appear with an asterisk (*). After pregnancy, once you get consent from your doctor, I suggest you do the towel abs exercises in Chapter 7 most days of the week to help guide those abdominal muscles back together again.

Now, at the same time, the body also starts producing elastin and relaxin, hormones that will relax and lengthen the ligaments (which connect bone to bone and help to keep joints stable) to make them ready for childbirth. You may notice that you seem to have a newfound flexibility. But it is important to strengthen the abdominals and obliques throughout pregnancy and beyond, because strong abdominals will counteract the lax ligaments, creating a more stable support system that will make the spine less vulnerable and ease any lower back issues.

The best way to work the transverse abdominal muscles is by exhaling and drawing your belly (abdominals) in toward the spine. Yes, this does get challenging as your pregnancy progresses, but to help you focus on where you need to be contracting, imagine that you're hugging the baby with your abs. On the flipside, if you hold your breath as you're going through the motion (which is quite common), you're not activating the deep abs and can cause your blood pressure to elevate. Not a good idea! So whatever you do, *breathe*!

Have you ever seen those big black support belts that wrap around your midsection? Well, this is exactly what these muscles do. However, some women do benefit from having a support belt around their hips as they get larger to compress the pelvic girdle for further support.

Your spinal placement is very important while performing any abdominal work. Our objective is to strengthen the abs in a way that helps us move better in the correct alignment. While performing abdominal exercises, you want to work from the natural placement of the spine (also called "neutral spine"). To find this position, stand up and think of the hip bones and the pubic bone making a triangle that is pointing downward (vertical), without overarching the lower spine. When you are lying on your back, the triangle is flat so that the pubic bone and hips are on one level plane. As you perform abdominal work, your aim is to start in a neutral spine and keep this position through the duration of the exercise. This requires the abdominals to work more effectively, holding the pelvis still as they stabilize the spine.

Exercising Your Pelvic Floor

Perhaps you're scratching your head as you read the title to this section, but if you've never thought about exercising your pelvic floor before, now is the time to start. One big change that you can't see during pregnancy is what happens to this area (and boy does it take a beating!).

The pelvic floor is made of three layers of muscle tissue that attach to the pubic bone, tailbone, and sit bones, and its job is to support the organs, provide sphincter control, and aid in orgasms. Before pregnancy the pelvic floor is relatively flat, but after pregnancy and childbirth it looks more like a sagging hammock. Problems that can result from this are urinary and fecal incontinence and pelvic pain and prolapse. Unfortunately, it doesn't just bounce back to normal without a little bit of help on your part. But if you strengthen this area *while* you're pregnant, you'll reduce the risk of these problems occurring later on.

Luckily, exercising this area doesn't require sneakers, a gym membership, or even breaking a sweat. You can strengthen the muscles in the base of the pelvis with "Kegel exercises" (named after the gynecologist who created them). You can do them while sitting, standing,

KEGEL EXERCISES

Quick Flicks
Squeeze the pelvic floor quickly and as hard as you can for 1 second, rest for 1 second. Repeat 10 times. Perform twice a day.

Long Holds
Squeeze the pelvic floor as hard as you can and hold for 5 seconds. Repeat 5 times, rest for 1 minute, and then do another set. You can do two sets 2 or 3 times a day at first, then progress slowly to do 10-second holds, with 10 repetitions, 2 or 3 times per day. Studies show that 30–45 10-second contractions per day can help to maintain pelvic floor strength.

or lying down (and no one will even know you're doing them, so you can exercise this area in your car, at a meeting, or over coffee with a friend!).

Here's how to do Kegels: If you were in public and suddenly felt the need to pass gas, your response would be to pull up and in at the rectum. A Kegel is when you pull the muscles of both the rectum and the vagina up inside your body. (I know this sounds weird, but imagine picking up marbles with your vagina and you'll get a sense of what I'm talking about.) To see if you are doing this correctly, place your hand on top of your pubic bone; when you tighten and draw in, you should feel the muscles lift toward your pubic bone and squeeze the openings shut. Just make sure you don't hold your breath while doing Kegels. This prevents you from pulling up properly—you'll know that you're doing this if your belly bulges while you contract your muscles. Counting out loud is a good way to avoid holding your breath. Also, beware of using other muscles like your butt, belly, or inner thighs to compensate—these areas should stay relaxed and your pelvis should stay still.

FIRST TRIMESTER EXERCISE PROGRAM

Most of the women on Team Mallett were pregnant with their second child and the rest worked full time, so even at this stage of their pregnancy, time was still a huge issue that had to be addressed. As a result, I created a plan that consists of a strength cardio circuit, core stability training, and flexibility exercises. Following this plan will allow you to maintain and build lean muscle mass and keep your body supple and healthy through your first trimester. As I mentioned above, you will return to these exercises in Phase I (7–19 weeks post-pregnancy). The women on Team Mallett loved that the workouts could be broken down into small chunks that they could squeeze into their unpredictable schedules. Here is what we will be focusing on and a quick snapshot of why it's so important:

Posture

During pregnancy your uterus expands up to 1,000 times its normal size (imagine that!), and this plus the added weight of your bulging belly can throw off your center of gravity and strain your back muscles. Strengthening postural muscles and stretching the tight hip flexors and hamstring muscles will bring you great relief. Doing so can even ward off back pain, sciatica (pain along the sciatic nerve, which runs from your lower back all the way down to your foot), and neck and shoulder pain. There's also an important aesthetic reason why you should keep these muscles strong. After all, who wants to look like a hunchback?

Core (Abs and Butt)

Abs and glutes play a huge part in keeping the pelvis stabilized and your pelvic floor strong through your pregnancy. These areas are also the first place to show water retention and cellulite. Working this area can help boost circulation and improve the appearance of those lovely pregnancy dimples.

Arms

Building strength in your arms is essential for when the baby arrives. Carrying 10–20 pounds a day will become the norm—and it's often more than that because of all the equipment the baby needs. (You'll be amazed to see how someone so small could require so much stuff!) Building strength in the upper body will protect you from common shoulder injuries that new mamas often experience.

Legs

Strong legs are definitely a plus when you're lugging the extra weight of the baby around for nine months (and when post-pregnancy you're toting your little one and all his or her belongings). Birthing squats also require a good amount of strength and endurance.

Stretching

Light total body stretching is also essential to keep your muscles supple as they start to stretch, making way for the arrival of the new baby. Muscles are tight during pregnancy from the constant shifting of your pelvic bones and from walking around with all that added weight. Your body also takes on a completely new shape in which your muscles will adapt by lengthening and tightening. Stretching is a miraculous yet easy way to relieve all those aches and pains.

Just a word of caution here: When you're pregnant, your body produces a hormone called relaxin, which helps make your joints looser so that your pelvis can open wider when it comes time for you to push out your baby. This is great news at delivery time, but for the nine months of

One of the not-so-pretty parts of this first trimester is good old morning sickness, which affects between 70 and 85 percent of pregnant women, according to the American College of Obstetricians and Gynecologists. When I got pregnant, I obviously knew that my stomach would expand to immense proportions and that I'd outgrow my favorite pair of jeans in a snap. But what I *didn't* know was that there would be a lot more going on in my belly than a growing baby.

Just weeks after my positive pregnancy test, I was incredibly queasy. Don't let the name "morning sickness" mislead you, since it can actually strike at any time of day or, as in my case, all day! Amazingly, this mild nausea and vomiting, which can come on at around 6 weeks and last up to 16 weeks, are actually a sign of a normal pregnancy. Experts aren't clear about what specifically causes morning sickness, but many have theories, including an increase in hormones, low blood sugar, increased sense of smell, excess stomach acid, and/or genetics.

During my first pregnancy, I was so sick that sometimes I wondered if I was actually suffering from the flu rather than pregnancy. It's a time when you're supposed to be jumping for joy, and all I could think about was finding the nearest bathroom. Exercise actually helped me feel better, which I know sounds strange because you're moving around and heating up the body during exercise. But I remember forcing myself to get on the elliptical machine, thinking that if I'm going to be sick anyway I might as well be sick doing something good for my body. Sure enough, exercise seemed to lift the nausea. My theory on this is that exercise helps your body to relax, gets valuable oxygen flowing, and improves circulation.

The other thing that worked for me was eating. Again, it sounds like the worst thing to do when you feel nauseous, but it helped. I didn't move an inch without having an arsenal of snacks in my pocket or purse so that when the slightest wave of queasiness came over me, I could fight it with my almonds or saltines! In fact, nutrition can play a vital role in combating morning sickness. Here are some other ideas that may help:

- Eat small, frequent meals, such as peanut butter on apples or celery, nuts, or cheese and crackers. Though food may be the last thing on your mind, the acid in an empty stomach may trigger nausea, and there's something about salty foods that may settle your stomach.
- Steer clear of odors. Your sense of smell is heightened during these nine months; even smells you normally love can make you feel sick. (I had to ban my husband from using his favorite after-shave, and I couldn't go near my mother if she used scented body lotion.) I prevented this by carrying a lemon wedge in a plastic baggie at all times. When I came across a bothersome smell, I'd take a whiff of its citrus scent and feel better on the spot.
- Keep snacks on your nightstand. Keeping some crackers or pretzels by your bed and nibbling on a few before getting up in the morning can help reduce stomach acids before you even move your body.
- Stay well hydrated by drinking plenty of water between meals or even sucking on ice chips or popsicles. However, limit fluids while eating, because some experts believe the combo of food sloshing around with liquid can make you feel sick.
- Peppermint and ginger teas are known to settle the stomach, or you can simply add lemon and ginger to your beverages. And though this sounds strange, one OB/GYN I know said that many of her patients find relief from hot chocolate.
- Though it's unclear why, anecdotal evidence suggests that watermelon can keep you from feeling queasy. If fresh watermelon isn't your thing, combine frozen pieces with lemon juice in a blender and then pour the pureed mixture into ice cube trays and freeze it. Enjoy your watermelon cubes several hours later.
- Try acupressure wristbands such as those used for seasickness (available at most drugstores). They have a small plastic button that puts pressure on a point on your wrist that's said to relieve queasiness.
- Allow plenty of time for rest and relaxation. Take regular catnaps, and don't underestimate the restorative impact of just 10 minutes of shut-eye or quiet time. Often simply reducing stress helped me alleviate my symptoms.

CAUTION: If vomiting becomes extreme, see your doctor as soon as possible. This may be a sign of a severe case of morning sickness called *hyperemesis gravidum* that occurs in less than 1 in 200 pregnancies and may require hospitalization.

pregnancy it means you may be more flexible than ever. Yes, for the first time in your life you may be able to do the splits, but don't even think of going there! If you let yourself stretch too far while pregnant, you can tear delicate tissue and cause injuries. Be sure to warm up before exercising, and even more importantly, take the time to cool down after you finish. Not only is this good for you physically, it's also a time to de-stress your mind, calm your nerves, and pamper yourself for a few private moments.

THINGS TO AVOID DURING PREGNANCY

- Stress. Pregnancy can be a stressful time for many women. Even if you're ecstatic about becoming a mom, you may also feel scared, be moody, or have a combo of many mixed emotions. Try and do what you can to relax because very high stress levels are thought to possibly contribute to low-birthweight or pre-term babies.
- Rodents. Mice, hamsters, guinea pigs, and others in this family can spread diseases that may harm your baby. If you have one of these rodents as a pet, keep it in a part of the house where you don't spend a lot of time or give it to a friend to babysit for nine months. Someone else should be cleaning the cage and feeding the pet throughout your pregnancy.
- Alcohol. Save the cocktails for your post-pregnancy celebration, because it's unclear what, if any, amount of alcohol is safe during pregnancy. Research shows that it can increase your baby's risk of birth defects even during the earliest weeks after conception.
- Saunas, hot tubs, and steam rooms. Their extremely high heat may be harmful for your growing and developing baby.
- Raw and undercooked meats. A parasite in both of these things can cause an infection called *toxoplasmosis*. It's also found on unwashed fruits and veggies (so scrub them before you eat), in cat litter boxes (have someone else change them), and anywhere outdoors where animal feces may be found.
- Fish that contains mercury. The Food and Drug Administration (FDA) and the Environmental Protection Agency (EPA) suggest that pregnant women, nursing moms, and young children avoid fish and shellfish that are high in mercury. Mercury can harm a fetus's or young child's developing nervous system. Don't eat shark, swordfish, king mackerel, or tilefish, and limit fish lower in mercury (like shrimp, canned light tuna, salmon, and catfish) to 12 ounces per week.
- Unpasteurized milk and milk products. These may contain listeria, a pathogen that can cause listeriosis, which can be harmful or even fatal to pregnant women and their babies. These include soft cheeses and other foods made with unpasteurized milk.

(For more information on foods and dietary supplements to avoid during pregnancy, see Chapter 5.)

Equipment Needed
This is what you'll need for the first-trimester exercises. For more detailed instructions on how to perform the exercises themselves, see Chapter 7, "Body After Baby Phase I: 7–19 Weeks Postpartum."

- Two sets of dumbbells, such as 3 pounds and 5 pounds (or 5 pounds and 8 pounds for those pregnant gals who've been working out for a while)
- Exercise band (available at most sporting goods stores, or www.spri.com)

CIRCUIT A

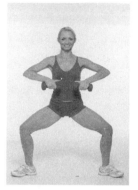 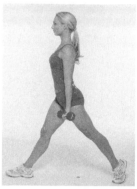 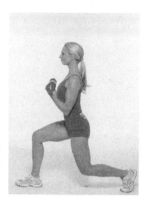

1. PLIÉ TO LUNGE WITH UPWARD ROW

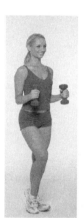 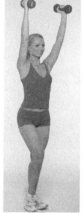 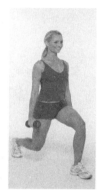

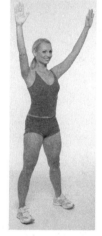 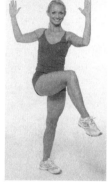

**2. LUNGE TO OVERHEAD PRESS
(STARTING IN BICEP HAMMER CURL)**

**CARDIO: KNEE TWIST ROTATION
FOR 60 SECONDS**

**3. CHAIR OR
COFFEE TABLE
PUSH-UPS
WITH LEG
EXTENSIONS**

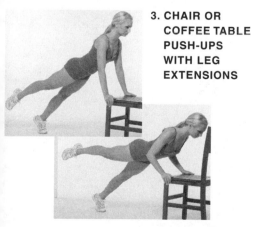

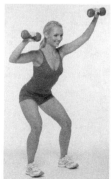 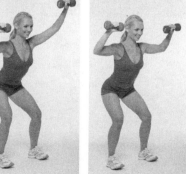

4. OVERHEAD PUNCHING

**CARDIO: REPEAT
KNEE TWIST
ROTATION FOR 60
SECONDS**

CIRCUIT B

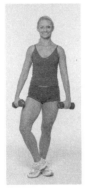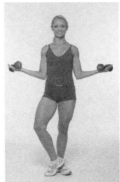

1. ANGLED BICEP CURLS

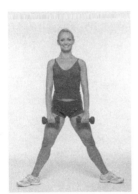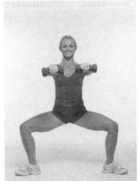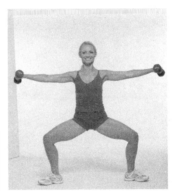

2. PLIÉ SQUAT WITH SHOULDER CIRCLES

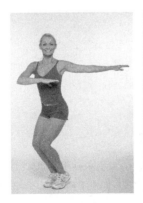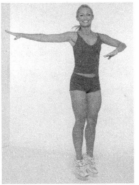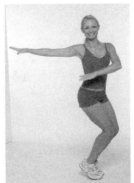

CARDIO: JUMP TWIST FOR 60 SECONDS

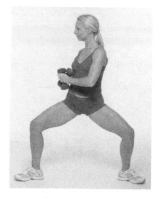
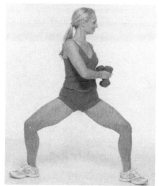

3. PLIÉ WITH ROTATION

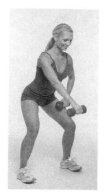
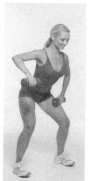
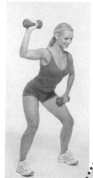

4. ROW WITH EXTERNAL ROTATION

CARDIO: REPEAT JUMP TWIST FOR 60 SECONDS

DID YOU KNOW?

Exercising during pregnancy may also help your future baby stay fit. A recent study in the *British Medical Journal* found that children whose moms were physically active during and after their pregnancies exercised more when they grew up than kids whose moms were pregnant couch potatoes.

TIPS TO AVOID AND QUELL HEARTBURN

1. Avoid caffeine, chocolate, acidic foods (such as citrus fruits and juices), and spicy, fried, or fatty foods.
2. Eat several small meals throughout the day instead of three large ones. Take your time eating, and chew thoroughly.
3. Chewing gum after eating will stimulate the salivary glands, which can help neutralize acid.
4. Don't eat close to bedtime. Give yourself 2 to 3 hours to digest before you lie down.
5. Sleep with your upper body propped up with pillows—this will keep your stomach acids where they belong.

CIRCUIT C

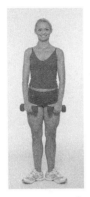 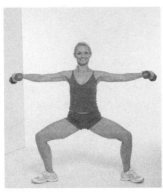 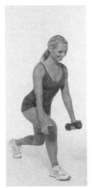 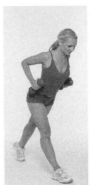

1. STEP PLIÉ TO SIDE (2 TO EACH SIDE) WITH SHOULDER RAISE

2. LUNGE WITH BENT-OVER ROW

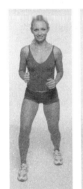 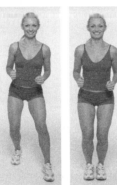 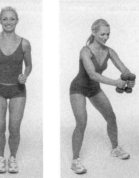 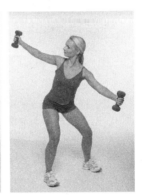 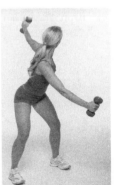

CARDIO: "OUT, OUT, IN IN" FOR 60 SECONDS

3. WINDMILL ROTATION

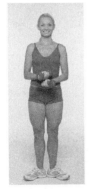 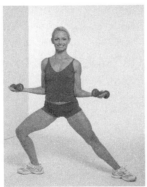

CARDIO: REPEAT "OUT, OUT, IN IN" FOR 60 SECONDS

4. ROTATOR CUFF WITH BICEPS IN PLIÉ POSITION

LOSE YOUR MOMMY TUMMY BLAST

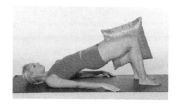 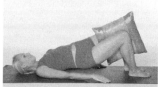 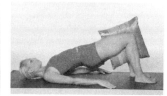

1. PELVIC BRIDGES WITH FIGURE EIGHTS*

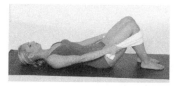 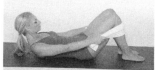

2. ABS TOWEL PULSE

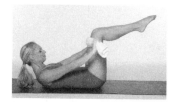 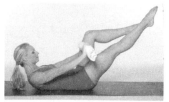

3. TOWEL-RESISTED SINGLE-LEG STRETCH

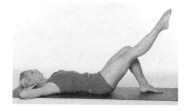

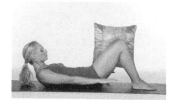 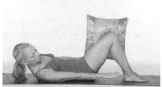

4. HEEL REACH

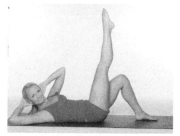

5. CHEST LIFT WITH SINGLE-LEG LIFT AND ROTATION

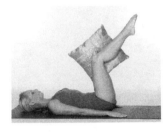
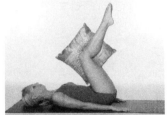

6. LOWER ABS CURL TILT

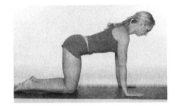
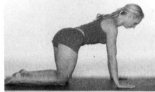
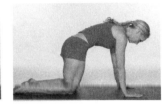

7. WAG THE TAIL 1*

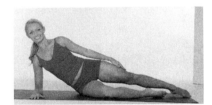
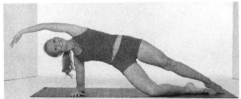

8. SIDE PLANK LIFTS*

MAMA BUTT BLAST

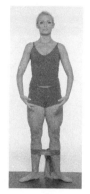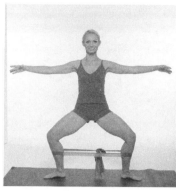

1. STEP SIDE GRAND PLIÉS

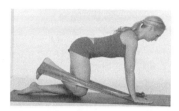

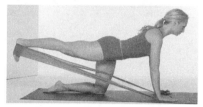

2. DONKEY KICK

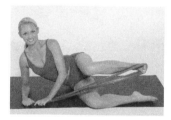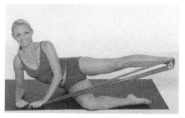

3. SIDE KICK WITH PULSES

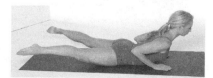

4. GLUTE BLASTERS

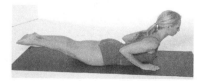

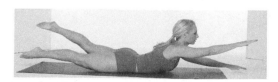

5. SWIMMING

6. HEEL BEATS

SUPER FIT MAMA FLEXIBILITY

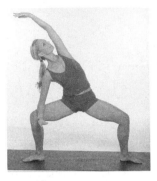

1. PLIÉS, SIDE ANGLE POSE

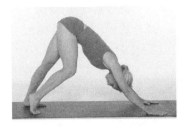

2. DOWNWARD DOG WITH WALKING

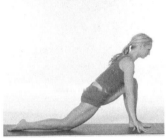

3. KNEELING HIP FLEXOR STRETCH

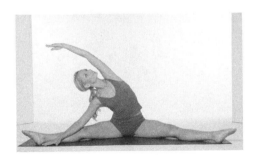

4. STRADDLE AND SIDE STRETCH

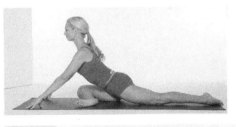

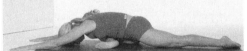

5. PIGEON POSE

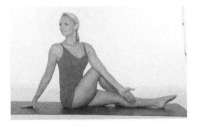

6. SEATED SPINAL ROTATION

Team Mallett Success Story

....

Anne Chapman, 34, Mission Viejo, CA

Lost

19 pounds

2 dress sizes

17 total inches

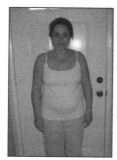 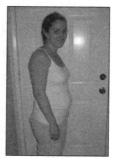 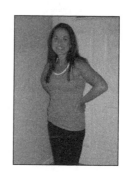

Before   After

• • • • •

Anne had three babies in three and a half years and gained between 25 and 35 pounds with each pregnancy. Though she lost some of the weight postpartum, she always started the next pregnancy with a few extra pounds. After her third child was born, Anne realized that she was finished being pregnant and that this was the body she'd have for the rest of her life. "That really scared me," she says. "After all, I no longer had the excuse that, 'I'm just going to get pregnant, so why diet now?'" Even scarier? Anne had been on numerous weight loss plans in the past without much success.

Before starting the Super Fit Mama plan, Anne felt so bad about her body that every time she went out she considered bringing along her newborn. "This way I could justify the extra weight because people would realize that I had just had a baby," says Anne. But a situation worse than going out was simply getting dressed. Anne's husband could sense her distress and would always try to say the "right" thing at those moments. "But after hearing him say, 'Don't worry about it, you just had a baby 8 weeks ago' for the eighth week in a row, I knew something had to be done or that statement would change from weeks to months!" says Anne. That's when she joined the Super Fit Mama plan.

To her surprise, the workouts were so easy to squeeze into her busy life that Anne was able to work out six days a week, and the variety kept her from getting bored. "The six-minute time frame is a dream for new moms or anyone with a tight schedule," she says. "It was nice to know that I could work out in separate sections or in one longer segment." The biggest surprise for her was that after years of hating crunches, she loved the ab workouts. "In the past, I've always felt like I had to do 100 crunches to make even a tiny difference," she says. "But with Tracey's simple ab segments, I finally have abs to be proud of."

"I finally know that it is doable to be fit despite my busy schedule and that I don't have to be content with a 'mommy body' that is pudgy but excusable because I have 3 kids," she says. Before starting the Super Fit Mama plan, Anne couldn't wait for her two older girls to take naps each day so that she could catch up on missed sleep herself. "But after starting the program, I no longer wanted to nap when the girls napped; I wanted to work out!"

After giving birth, Anne's body image was "horrible." Plus, she was exhausted all the time and still had to take care of two older children and keep up her house. Today, she has energy and confidence to burn. "Tracey's program gave me time to think about myself—not my three young girls or my husband—and work for a goal that was mine and mine alone!"

TEAM MALLETT FEELS YOUR PAIN

"To alleviate low back pain in the beginning of pregnancy, I took a warm bath and did pelvic tilts, which helped to relieve the pressure. (Eventually it went away with the natural progression of pregnancy.) Also, smelling peppermint and natural vanilla helped to alleviate my severe first-trimester nausea."—Andrea Frye

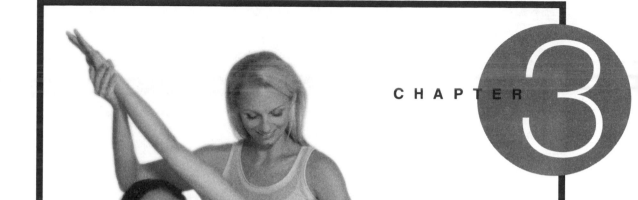

CHAPTER 3

SECOND TRIMESTER FITNESS
The Honeymoon Phase

GET OUT THOSE CHAMPAGNE GLASSES, FILL 'EM WITH sparkling grape juice, and toast to the fact that you're a third of the way through this nine-month adventure! Even better, it's likely that the worst morning sickness is behind you. Typically around week 13 those queasy, crazy days of the first trimester come to an end—and sometimes they do so seemingly overnight. Now you'll enter what is called the "honeymoon phase" of pregnancy. By the fourth month of pregnancy, you've probably started showing and see a rounder reflection in the mirror. Finally, your body is beginning to advertise that you're indeed a mama-in-the-making.

YOUR BABY

- By 13 weeks your baby is the size of a medium shrimp.
- By 16 weeks your baby is the size of an avocado.
- By 18 weeks your baby is about the size of a bell pepper.
- By 21 weeks your baby is about as long as a carrot.
- By 23 weeks your baby weighs as much as a large mango.

For those of you who are lucky enough to be having a totally symptom-free pregnancy, it will probably get even easier for you now. For the rest of us, things do get better. I was now able to make it through the day without throwing up or taking a nap. I had loads of energy, and best of all, my middle-of-the-night bathroom trips went from four to two, so I actually slept a little better. It truly felt like a reason to celebrate. However, a word of caution for those of you who start to feel like Superwoman. After three months of feeling totally out of control with your body, it's easy to go over the top taking on all the tasks that you dreamed about doing over the past few months. Remember, listen to your body!

But now that you're feeling better, it's a great time to work out, and later in this chapter I'll show you exercises designed with a typical second trimester in mind. They will not only make you feel better through the next three months but will also get you in shape for the physical feat of labor and childbirth. Exercise at the time of day when you feel your best (this varies from person to person). Of course, check with your doctor before starting any prenatal exercise program. Keep in mind, too, that your joints are looser during pregnancy, so be careful that you don't stretch yourself too far or you will cause yourself injuries. And be sure to warm up your body before exercising and cool down after you finish.

Finally, if you experience any of the following, *stop exercising immediately* and call your doctor or midwife:

1. **Vaginal bleeding**
2. **Muscle weakness**
3. **Calf pain or swelling**
4. **Dizziness**
5. **Headache**
6. **Overheating**
7. **Pain or heavy pressure in the pubic bone area**
8. **Shortness of breath**
9. **Cramps**
10. **Chest pain**
11. **Severe nausea**
12. **Leakage of amniotic fluid**

There may be days when you'll only want to work out for 12 minutes instead of doing the full 32-minute program, and others when you'll only be able to eke out 6 minutes. But even doing 6 minutes of activity will make you feel better than doing nothing at all, and you'll still reap some benefits both physically and mentally. Some days you might just do light stretches and walk around the block. Other times you might squeeze in mini-fitness breaks by practicing the all-important Kegels for the good old pelvic floor muscles. And some days, the most exercise you'll get is walking from the couch to the bathroom. (Though I peed so often that I considered clocking my steps with a pedometer!)

The key is not to beat yourself up if you are having a down day and can't find the time or energy to do the full exercise program. Every little bit of exercise will eventually help you achieve your goal of wellness. Remember, it's not just about your body; now you're responsible for another body, your baby! Now that's a major inspiration.

> Voluntarily contract the pelvic floor during pliés, squats, attitudes, clams, and hip adductor exercises. This is a great way to complete the recommended amount of daily Kegel exercises.

COMMON PHYSICAL CHANGES IN THE SECOND TRIMESTER

- **You may experience** diastasis recti, a separation of the abdominals that forces the connective tissue in the center of the abdominal muscles, called the *linea alba*, to stretch. It usually heals on its own post-pregnancy.
- **You may develop** *linea nigra*, a dark brown line that runs down the center of the abdominal area of some women during pregnancy. It can look strange, but no worries; it's temporary and will fade away after pregnancy. How long it sticks around varies from woman to woman and is affected by whether you breastfeed.
- **Back pain** is one of the most common discomforts for moms-to-be. It's the result of your uterus expanding up to 1,000 times its pre-pregnancy size and the added weight that changes your center of gravity and posture. All of this can strain your back muscles. Some ways to get relief: pregnancy massages (or rubdowns from your partner), sitting in chairs with good back support, not standing on your feet for long periods of time, and performing the core-strengthening and flexibility segments on most days of the week. Also, try to maintain proper posture. Many women tend to allow their low backs to sway or arch as their bellies grow bigger and drop forward. Try to keep your lower back neutral by tucking your tailbone under and contracting the abs.
- **Sciatica** is pain and/or numbness and tingling that radiates from your buttocks down the back of your leg to your knee (that is, along the sciatic nerve, the longest nerve of your body). During pregnancy, it is often the result of postural changes that occur as your belly grows that can cause spasm of the muscles of the buttock and then compress and irritate the sciatic nerve. A heating pad applied to the lower back and buttocks, or massage, yoga, and stretching, may alleviate the pain. So will performing the glute and hamstring stretches in the flexibility segment above. Be sure to tell your prenatal doctor if you are experiencing sciatic pain so that you may be referred to physical therapy for treatment.
- **Feeling off balance** is common during the second trimester, thanks to your ever-expanding belly changing your center of gravity. Performing regular abdominal work like the exercises in the core-conditioning segment in this chapter will keep your center strong and improve your posture, which in turn will improve your balance. Of course, if you feel unsteady while doing certain exercises, hold onto a chair, countertop, or even your mate, if needed.
- **Carpal tunnel syndrome** is marked by pain, numbness, tingling, or burning in your fingers, palm, or wrist or radiating up your arm. Some people say their fingers feel swollen even though they don't look like they are. It can occur as the result of repetitive motions like those experienced by people who work with computer keyboards at their jobs, but during pregnancy it is often the result of swelling in the wrist, which compresses the median nerve. Stretches, wrist braces (available at the drugstore), and not sleeping on your hands can help. See "Other Helpful Stretches" below for some relief.
- **Leg cramps** are oh-so-painful muscle contractions that last for just a few minutes. They often happen at night and are common during the second and third trimesters. Stretching your legs, walking around a bit, or massaging the affected area can soothe them. See "Other Helpful Stretches" below for some relief.
- **Round ligament pain,** pain in the pelvic area due to the stretching and thickening of the round ligaments that surround your uterus, usually begins in the second trimester. It can feel like a dull ache or a brief, stabbing pain roughly along the bikini line area. See "Other Helpful Stretches" below for some relief.

SECOND TRIMESTER WORKOUT PLAN

You may now find that you have a new burst of energy and that you're ready to start working out after a few months of feeling lethargic, weak, and possibly seasick! All of the following exercises have been modified or replaced from the previous chapter to be suitable and safe while avoiding second trimester contraindications.

For the second trimester workout plan, see Table 3.1. It consists of the following:

3 Cardio Strength Training Circuits
1 Super Fit Mama Core Conditioning Segment
1 Super Fit Mama Flexibility Segment

TABLE 3.1: SECOND TRIMESTER SAMPLE WORKOUT PLAN

	MONDAY	TUESDAY	WEDNESDAY	THURSDAY	FRIDAY	SATURDAY
Circuits	*		*		*	
Core	*		*		*	
Flexibility	*	*	*	*	*	*
Cardio						
20–30 Minutes		*		*		*

SECOND TRIMESTER EXERCISE DON'TS:

- Avoid working out in the supine position (lying on your back). The increased weight of the baby can inhibit blood flow and oxygen to the fetus. Make some of your favorite exercises safer and easier by adding pillows so that you're elevating your head above your heart. (Though always check with an expert if you're not sure an exercise can be safely done this way.) If you do lay on your back, even if you feel totally comfortable, it is still not recommended to stay there for more than 5 minutes.
- Avoid inversion poses like yoga shoulder and headstands, or the Pilates jackknife, double leg lower lifts, and rollover.
- Perform the downward dog only with caution. This is a popular yoga pose in which the practitioner begins on his or her hands and knees, and then raises the hips toward the ceiling to form an upside-down "V" shape to get a full-body stretch. The safety of this pose during pregnancy is somewhat controversial among experts, but here's my theory: Any exercise where your head is lower than your heart should be practiced only in moderation after the first trimester, because the additional blood volume of pregnancy can lead to nausea. If you want to do the downward dog, don't hold the position for extended periods of time, and modify it by keeping your knees bent and your heels lifted off the floor to reduce stress on your lower spine. Your arms should also be positioned a little further apart than in your regular practice. The modification means that your body weight will now be supported predominantly by your upper body to reduce compression of your abdomen.

Note: If you're starting to experience lower back pain, I recommend that you perform the core and the flexibility segment 5–6 times a week. You will gain more strength and flexibility to help ease the pain and prevent it from getting worse.

SECOND TRIMESTER CARDIO STRENGTH TRAINING CIRCUIT

Time: 6 to 8 minutes per circuit segment, not including the warm-up

How to: Perform each exercise once using the recommended set of weights. Repeat if you'd like to do another set. I've suggested a number of reps for each exercise, but if you are just starting out, you may start lower and work up to these targets.

You'll need: Two sets of dumbbells, a chair, and a pillow or rolled-up towel. (For each exercise I've indicated which set of dumbbells to use with the terms "Lighter" and "Heavier." These could be 3-lb. and 5-lb. weights, or, if you're just starting out, you might choose to use 1-lb. and 3-lb. weights instead, or 2-lb. and 4-lb. weights. If one set seems too heavy for you, go with a lighter set until you are ready to move up.)

CIRCUIT A

Warm-up: March in place for 1 or 2 minutes, making large, slow, rhythmic movements. Circle your arms forward and back while taking deep breaths.

1. Triceps stationary lunges

Muscles targeted: Quads, hamstrings, glutes, and triceps

Reps: 15 on each leg

Weights: Lighter

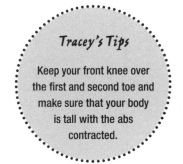

Tracey's Tips

Keep your front knee over the first and second toe and make sure that your body is tall with the abs contracted.

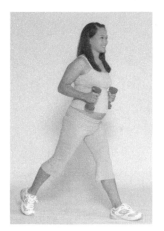 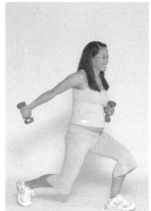

A. Start standing tall with your left leg forward and right leg behind you. Make sure both feet are facing forward with the back foot resting on a toe, and that your left arm is bent behind you with your right hand resting on your right thigh.

B. Exhale and bend both legs into a lunge position as you extend your elbow, contracting the back of the upper arm (triceps). Inhale, extend both knees, and bend the elbow back to start position.

Modification: If you're having problems with your balance, hold onto a chair for support, or follow the modification in the third trimester.

2. Attitude side lift with shoulder raise

Muscles targeted: Quads, glutes, and shoulders (deltoids)

Reps: 10 on each leg

Weights: Lighter

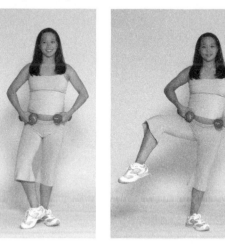
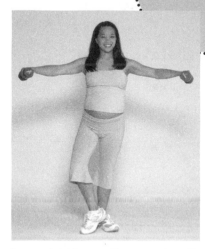

A. Stand with your legs turned out at the hips and your right leg resting on a toe, then place your hands on your hips.

B. Exhale and lift your right leg off the floor with knee bent, leading with the knee to the side of the body. Inhale and lower the leg back to start position.

C. Exhale and lift the arms to the side of the body to shoulder height, leading with the elbows. Lower arms then alternate the leg lift and the lateral arm raise for 10 reps before switching to the other side.

Modification: If this is difficult for you, do not lift the leg as high as pictured, or follow the third trimester modification by holding onto a chair for support.

Note: Place weights on the floor.

Cardio:

Knee raises for 60 seconds.

Step onto the right foot and lift your left knee toward your chest. At the same time, reach your hands forward at shoulder height and then pull back to the waist as you bend your elbows.

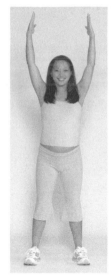
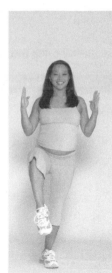

3. Plié and pelvic tilt with "V" to "W" arms

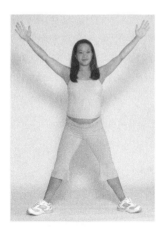

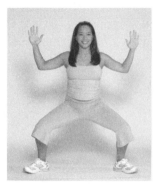

Muscles targeted: Quads, hamstrings, abs, pelvic floor, shoulders, and mid to upper back

Reps: 20

Weights: Lighter

A. Start with your legs a little further than hip-width apart, legs turned out at the hips and toes pointing out to the corners of the room. Bend your knees into a plié position to the point where you feel your thighs start to work. Your knees should be over your first and second toes. Place your arms over your head in a wide "V" position, pulling your shoulders down toward your pelvis.

B. Exhale and tilt your pelvis forward by contracting your abdominals and drawing your pubic bone up toward your belly button. At the same time, draw your elbows down toward your hips into a "W" position by contracting the lats (sides of the back). Then move the pelvis back to neutral (start position), extending the arms back to a "V" position. Do 20 reps then perform 20 little pulses (small movements with the pelvis) before extending the legs.

Tracey's Tips

Draw the pelvis slightly underneath you so that you are not overarching your back. Keep the toes over the knees and the weight on your heels.

4. Squat row

Muscles targeted: Quads, hamstrings, glutes, and mid to upper back

Reps: 15

Weights: Heavier

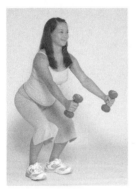 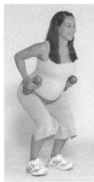

A. Start with your legs shoulder-width apart and your hands by your sides. Bend both knees into a squat, resting your weight in your heels and reaching your arms out in front of your body at shoulder height with palms facing toward each other.

B. Exhale, squeeze your shoulder blades together, and draw your elbows back behind your body into a rowing position. Inhale and extend the arms and legs, then repeat. Do a total of 15 reps.

Tracey's Tips

Keep your weight back in the heels and your body slightly pitched forward hinging from the waist. Your abs must always be contracted to support your midsection.

Note: Place weights on the floor.

Cardio:

Repeat knee raises for 60 seconds.

Cooldown: Walk or march in place for a few minutes to bring your heart rate down slightly before moving on to the next circuit.

CIRCUIT B

1. Pliés with angle bicep curls

Muscles targeted: Quads, hamstrings, glutes, biceps, and shoulders

Reps: 20

Weights: Heavier

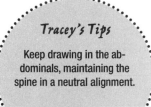

Tracey's Tips

Keep drawing in the abdominals, maintaining the spine in a neutral alignment.

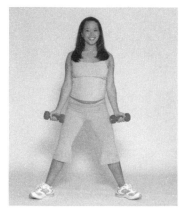 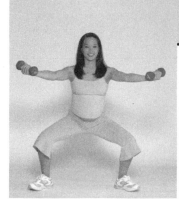 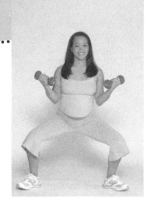

A. Start with your feet shoulder-width apart, turned out at the hips with the toes pointing out to the corners of the room. Bend your arms slightly at the sides of your hips with your palms facing upward.

B. Bend both legs so that your knees are over your toes while you lift your arms up to shoulder height, then extend your legs as you lower the arms back down.

C. Next time bend the elbows into a bicep curl. Alternate the arm lift with the bicep curl.

2. Squat with posterior deltoid flies

Muscles targeted: Quads, hamstrings, glutes, and posterior deltoids (back of the shoulders)

Reps: 15

Weights: Lighter

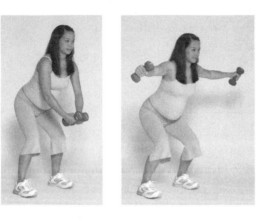

A. Start with the feet shoulder-width apart, arms slightly rounded in front of the body with palms facing inward and your body slightly pitched forward from the waist.

B. Bend your knees as you shift your weight back into the heels and lift your arms out to the sides, leading with the elbows and drawing your shoulder blades together.

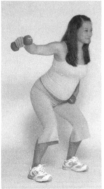

Modification: Perform one arm at a time to decrease the load. Keep the abs pulled in so you don't twist your spine.

Note: Place weights on the floor.

Cardio:

Traveling sideways, step touch for 60 seconds.

Step two-step touches to the right, opening the arms out to the side at shoulder height, and then as you bring your legs together take the arms down, up, and down. Repeat to the left side, keeping your knees slightly bent at all times.

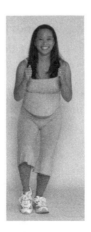
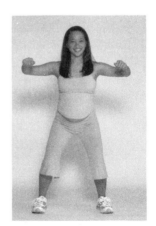

3. Triceps dips

Muscles targeted: Triceps

Reps: 15

Weights: None

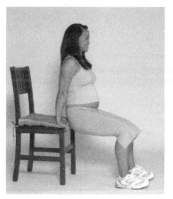 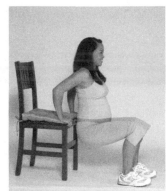

A. Start by sitting on the edge of a chair with your elbows bent, hands resting on the corner of the seat with fingers facing forward, knees bent hip-width apart, and spine in a neutral position.

B. Lift your hips off the seat and inhale as you bend your elbows as far as you can without hiking your shoulders toward your ears. Exhale and extend the elbows, then repeat. This is a slow and controlled movement.

Modification: Refrain from doing this exercise if you suffer from carpal tunnel syndrome. Instead, perform a standing tricep extension (see third trimester modification).

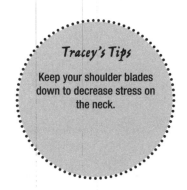

Tracey's Tips

Keep your shoulder blades
down to decrease stress on
the neck.

4. Lateral side leg lift with shoulders and biceps

Muscles targeted: Shoulders, biceps, and glutes

Reps: 15 on each leg

Weights: Lighter

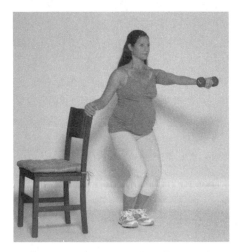

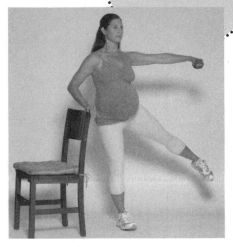

A. Stand beside a chair with your legs together, knees slightly bent, and your right (outside) arm resting by your side. The inside hand is resting on the chair for support. Exhale and extend the right (outside) leg out to the side off the floor just below hip height. Make sure your toe is facing forward. At the same time extend your right arm out to the side in a lateral shoulder raise, leading with elbow.

B. Bring your lower leg back into start position, then extend the arm forward to shoulder height with the palm facing downward. Do 15 reps on the same side, then repeat on the other side.

Modification: If lifting the leg is uncomfortable for you, do not lift it but simply extend it to a point on the floor.

Note: Place weights on the floor

Cardio:

Traveling sideways, step touch for 60 seconds.

Cooldown: Walk or march in place for a few minutes to bring your heart rate down slightly before moving on to the next circuit.

CIRCUIT C

1. Plié to heel rise

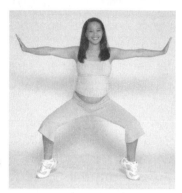

Muscles targeted: Glutes, hamstrings, quads, and abs

Reps: 10–15

Weights: None

A. Start with your legs a little further than shoulder-width apart with your toes pointing to the corners of the room and your legs turned out at the hips. Extend your arms out to the side at shoulder height with your hands flexed.

B. Bend both knees into a plié position, lift both heels off the floor, then lower the heels and extend the knees. Repeat 10–15 times.

Modification: Do only pliés without lifting the heels off the floor if the heel rise is difficult.

Tracey's Tips

Draw the abs in toward the spine as if you're hugging the baby with your abs. This will take the strain out of the lower back. Make sure your knees are over your toes and your legs are turned out at the hips, not the knees.

Keep the shoulder blades pulled down and the spine tall throughout the arm circles.

2. Arm circles

Muscles targeted: Shoulders, upper back, quads, hamstrings, and glutes

Reps: 10 circles forward and 10 circles back

Weights: None

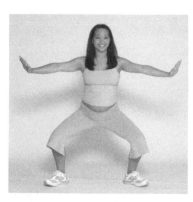

A. Stand with your legs a little further than shoulder-width apart, toes pointing to the corners of the room and legs turned out at the hips, and arms extended out to the side, shoulder height, with hands flexed.

B. Bend both knees into a plié position, circle the arms forward in small circles for 10 reps, then repeat in the opposite direction.

Cardio:

Hamstring curl for 60 seconds (no weights).

Step to the left, then bend the right knee, bringing the heel toward the butt, and bend your elbows at the side of your body. Repeat, alternating the legs for 60 seconds. Keep both knees bent at all times and focus on squeezing the hamstrings as you bring the heel to the butt.

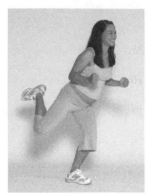

3. Yoga chair with heel rise

Muscles targeted: Glutes, hamstrings, quads, and calves

Reps: 15

Weights: None

Tracey's Tips

Press the weight into your heels during the squat and extend the upper spine by drawing your shoulder blades down toward the hips.

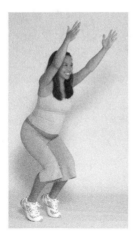

A. Start with your feet hip-width apart and your arms by your sides. Bend both knees into a squat while lifting both arms overhead in line with your ears. Tilt the pelvis under by drawing in your abdominals.

B. Rise up onto your toes and then lower your heels and extend your knees, bringing the arms back to the sides of your body.

Modification: Bend the knees into the squat, but then return to the start position instead of lifting the heels.

4. Hitch a ride

Muscles targeted: Mid to upper back, shoulders, glutes, quads, and hamstrings

Reps: 15 with 10 pulses

Weights: None

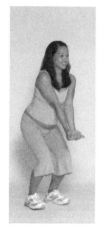 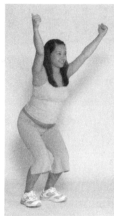

A. Start with your feet hip-width apart and knees bent with your weight in your heels. Your arms are straight in front of the body with your palms facing upward and your thumbs extended.

B. Exhale and lift your arms into a "V" position, leading with the thumbs, as you extend the spine, then bring your arms back to the start position. Repeat for 15 reps, staying in a squat position, then add tiny pulses (small up and down movements) for 10 reps.

Cardio:

Repeat hamstring curl for 60 seconds (no weights).

Cooldown: Walk in place for a few minutes to bring your heart rate back down to a normal pace. Breathe deeply.

Tracey's Tips

As you lift your arms over your head, try to keep the shoulder blades drawing down and back so that you don't create stress in the neck and shoulders.

SUPER FIT MAMA CORE STRENGTHENING

The second trimester is a good time to start monitoring your abdominal separation with this simple test. If you show signs of developing diastasis recti, a condition that involves a separation in the rectus abdominus muscles, you will need to take some precautions.

To see if you have a separation, place a pillow diagonally against the back of a chair and sit on a slight incline, with your upper spine resting on the pillow, knees bent and toes pointing forward. Place your fingers just above your belly button, then exhale and lift your head, neck, and shoulders off the chair as you look down toward your belly. Repeat these steps with your fingers below the belly button. If you can feel a separation of two to three fingers or more, be cautious when doing core-strengthening exercises. Below, the exercises that are safe to do with diastasis recti are marked with an asterisk (*). (This rule is used throughout the book, but only pertains to the core-strengthening exercises.)

Time: 6 to 8 minutes.

How to: Perform one set of each of the following exercises.

You'll need: Three pillows and a rolled-up towel or exercise band.

Note: An asterisk (*) denotes that an exercise is safe to perform even if you have diastasis recti. This rule only applies in the core-strengthening segment.

YOUR BODY

- By week 16 your nausea should be subsiding.
- Between weeks 16 and 20 you can feel your baby move for the first time.
- You will start to show the classic "bump" during this trimester: It's time to get the maternity clothes out!
- Your abdominal muscles may start to separate, so it's also time to start monitoring your abs.
- You will feel more energetic and in the land of the living.
- You will average a 1–2 pound weight gain per week.

1. Wag the tail version 1*

Muscles targeted: Abdominals and pelvic floor

Reps: 8 on each side

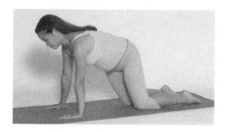 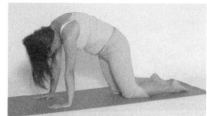

A. Position yourself on your hands and knees. Make sure your hands are shoulder-width apart and directly under your shoulders and your knees are stacked under your hips.

B. Move your hips to the right side as if you were a dog wagging your tail, then draw your abs in and do a pelvic tilt. Return to center and then repeat to the other side.

2. Cat pillow squeeze*

Muscles targeted: Inner thighs and pelvic floor

Reps: 10

Tracey's Tips

As you do the pelvic tilt, contract the pelvic floor. Keep the stress out of your upper body by pulling your shoulders away from your ears and not sinking in between the shoulder blades.

Imagine that you're drawing your knees together, focus on the inner thighs doing all the work, and contract the pelvic floor.

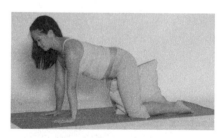 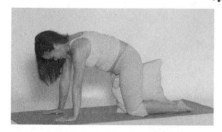

A. Position yourself on your hands and knees, with legs hip-width apart and a pillow between your inner thighs. Make sure your shoulders are over your hands and your hips are over your knees.

B. Squeeze the pillow and tilt your pelvis, drawing your abdominals in toward the spine and your pubic bone toward the belly button, and pull up the pelvic floor like an elevator. Inhale and return to the neutral position. Repeat 10 times.

3. Knee abdominal swing

Muscles targeted: Abdominals, pelvic floor, glutes, and upper body

Reps: 10 on each side

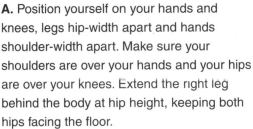

A. Position yourself on your hands and knees, legs hip-width apart and hands shoulder-width apart. Make sure your shoulders are over your hands and your hips are over your knees. Extend the right leg behind the body at hip height, keeping both hips facing the floor.

B. Exhale and draw the abdominals in as you imagine that you're hugging your baby. Bend the right knee toward the belly and curve the spine as your pubic bone moves toward your belly button in a pelvic tilt. Inhale and extend the leg back behind the body. Repeat for 10 reps before moving to the other leg.

4. Knee lifts with leg extension (pillow version on the floor)

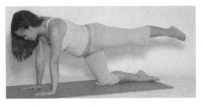

Note: If you have diastasis recti (separation in your abdominals), discussed above, skip this exercise and instead do the modification (chair version).

Muscles targeted: Abdominals and quads

Reps: 10 on each leg

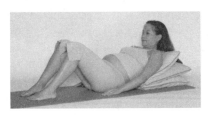

A. Place your upper back on three pillows to create an incline so that your head is elevated above your heart, and bend your knees so that your heels are level with your sit bones.

B. Extend your arms out to your sides and lift your right leg up so that it is level with your left knee and slightly bent.

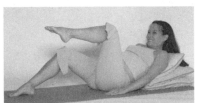

C. Inhale and extend the leg straight out, then exhale, contract the abs, and bend the knee toward the chest. Do 10 reps, then bend your knee and lower your leg to the floor before repeating to the other side.

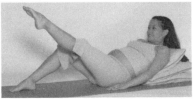

Modification: Knee lifts with leg extension (chair version)*

Muscles targeted: Abdominals and pelvic floor

Reps: 10

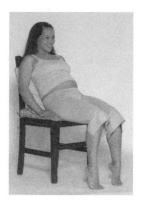 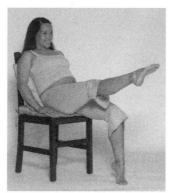 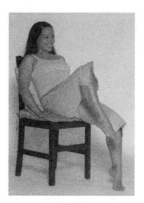

A. Place a pillow at a diagonal resting on the back of the chair. Sit down with your tailbone a few inches from the end of the chair and your upper body against the back so that your body is on an incline. Bend your knees, with your feet resting on the floor and your toes pointing forward. Lift the right leg off the floor so that your leg is extended straight out in front of you, at hip height.

B. Inhale and bend your right knee toward the chest, then exhale and extend the leg back out to the start position. Do 10 reps, then bend your knee and lower your foot back to the floor before repeating to the other side.

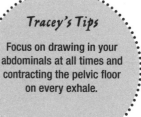

Tracey's Tips

Focus on drawing in your abdominals at all times and contracting the pelvic floor on every exhale.

5. Plank forearm knee drops

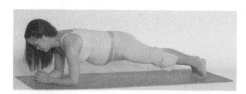

Muscles targeted: Abdominals

Reps: 10–15

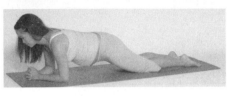

A. Begin in a plank position, face down and body parallel to the floor, balancing on your forearms with your elbows bent. Your shoulders should be directly in line with your elbows, and your legs are extended with your toes turned under so that you're also balancing on the balls of your feet. You should be in a straight line from the crown of your head to your heels.

B. Inhale and drop the knees towards the floor without moving the upper body, then exhale and lift the knees off the floor. Complete 10–15 reps. If you want to challenge yourself a little further, hold the pose for 20 seconds.

Tracey's Tips

When you drop your knees down to the floor, your body should be in a diagonal line from the crown of the head to the knees.

Keep the shoulder blades pulling toward the hips, especially on the supporting arm, to avoid tension in the shoulder and neck. Avoid overarching the back by keeping the abs contracted at all times.

6. T-stand with oblique contractions*

Muscles targeted: Obliques, lats, glutes, and legs

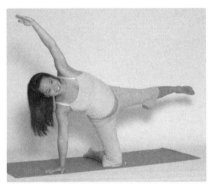
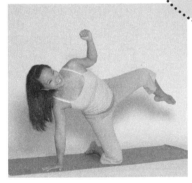

A. Start by sitting on your right hip with your knees bent and your right arm straight, resting on the floor. Your left arm is by the side of the left hip. Exhale and lift the hips off the floor, extend the top (left) leg straight out to the side, and reach the left arm up and over the body into a side stretch and hold for a couple of seconds.

B. Exhale and bend the left leg toward your upper body as you bend the left arm toward the knee, contacting the obliques. Extend the leg and arm back to the same position, then repeat.

Modification: Hold the T-stand without any movement (see third trimester modification*).

Reps: 8–10 on each side

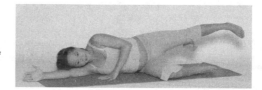

7. Side line butt zap*

Muscles targeted: Glutes

Reps: 20 on each leg

A. Start by lying on your right hip with your right leg bent and the left leg extended straight out at hip height. Extend your right arm and rest your right ear on your bicep, and place your left hand in front of the chest on the floor for support.

B. Turn the toes on your left foot down to the floor and lift the leg up and down for 10 reps, then turn the toes upward and do another 10 reps.

Tracey's Tips

Keep your hips stacked on top of each other facing forward at all times. Imagine your body being supported by a wall behind you. There should be little or no movement in the torso.

SUPER FIT MAMA FLEXIBILITY

Time: 6 to 8 minutes.

How to: Perform each exercise and hold the stretch for the recommended amount of time. If you're feeling really tight, you can hold the stretch a little longer. Remember not to push your newfound flexibility from the pregnancy hormone relaxin; go only to a place that feels comfortable and not painful.

You'll need: Pillow.

1. Sitting glute stretch on the floor

Muscles targeted: Glutes and the piriformis

Hold for 30 seconds on each side

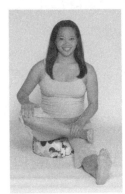

A. Sit tall on top of a pillow with your right leg extended in front of you and your foot flexed. Place your left foot on top of your right knee and turn the thigh out at the hip. Place your left hand on your left knee and your right hand on your right thigh.

B. Hinge forward from your hips to the point where you feel a comfortable stretch in your glutes. Extend forward from your sternum, lengthening out your lower spine.

2. Kneeling hip flexor stretch

Muscles targeted: Hip flexors and quads

Hold for 30 seconds on each leg

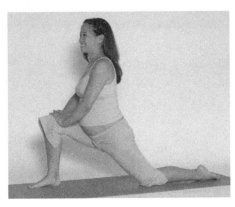

A. Start in a lunge position with your right leg in front of you and your left knee resting on the floor. Your right knee should be directly above the toes.

B. Rest your hands on the right knee and straighten your spine, breathing deeply as you hold the stretch. Switch legs and repeat.

Modification: Place your hands on either side of your foot, or, if balance is an issue, use a chair for support (see third trimester modification).

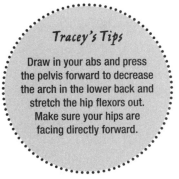

Tracey's Tips

Draw in your abs and press the pelvis forward to decrease the arch in the lower back and stretch the hip flexors out. Make sure your hips are facing directly forward.

3. Sitting hamstring stretch

Muscles targeted: Hamstrings

Hold for 30 seconds on each leg

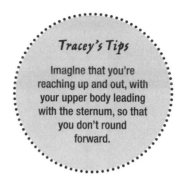

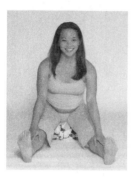

A. Sit tall on the pillow, bend your right leg turned out at the hip, and extend your left leg slightly out on a diagonal to make room for your belly.

B. Place your hands on either side of the left leg and hinge forward from your hips, leading with the sternum while extending the upper spine. Repeat on the other side.

Modification: This stretch can be done in a chair (see third trimester).

4. Butterfly

Muscles targeted: Inner thighs

Hold for 30 seconds

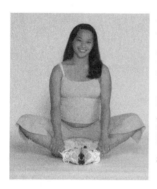

A. Sit down on the floor or on a pillow and place the soles of your feet together with your knees wide and out to the sides. Hold onto your shins, place your elbows on top of the inner thighs to create gentle resistance, then open the hips a little further.

B. Leading with the sternum, hinge your torso forward from the hips and hold, gently trying to increase the stretch in the hips.

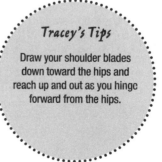

5. Spine stretch with thumb pulses

Muscles targeted: Mid to upper back and hamstrings

Reps: 8 with 8 pulses each

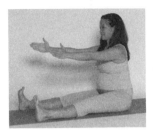 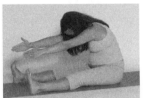 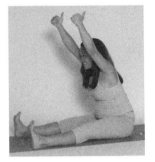

A. Sit tall on the floor or on a pillow (the pillow is especially good if you have tight hamstrings), extend your legs in front of you shoulder-width apart, and extend your arms out in front of you at shoulder height.

B. Exhale, contract the abs, and curl up and over, as if you're going up and over a big beach ball as you reach forward toward your feet.

C. Inhale and extend the spine as you move your arms so that your biceps are by your ears. With thumbs on top, gently pulse the thumbs up to the ceiling as you draw your shoulder blades down the back to work on the mid to upper back. Exhale and curl forward, up over your beach ball, to return to the start position.

Tracey's Tips

Imagine that you have a beach ball sitting in front of your torso as you reach up and over toward the feet, drawing in the abdominals tight.

Hold for just 15 seconds at first and work up to 45 seconds as you develop more stamina.

6. Birthing squat

Muscles targeted: Quads, hamstrings, glutes, and pelvic floor

Hold for 15–45 seconds

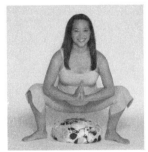

A. Start with your legs hip-width apart and bend your knees into a squat so that your hips are a few inches off the floor or resting on a pillow for support.

B. Shift your weight to your heels and place your hands together in a prayer position in front of the chest as you press your elbows against the inner thighs to gently open the hips. Extend the knees back to a standing position.

Modification: Sit tall on the edge of a chair with your legs bent and turned out at the hips (see third trimester).

7. Side angle pose

Muscles targeted: Glutes, inner thighs, hamstrings, quads, and obliques

Hold for 20–30 seconds on each side

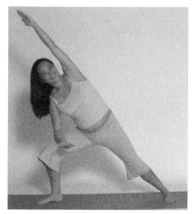

A. Start with your legs a little further than shoulder-width apart, turned out from the hips, with the toes pointing out to the corners of the room. Bend your legs so that your knees are over your toes and place your right forearm on your right thigh. Reach the left arm and stretch your body to the right, using your right forearm as resistance to open the hips further. Look up toward the inside of the left arm. Hold this pose for 20–30 seconds, then switch sides.

Modification: Sit on a chair for support while performing the stretch.

Tracey's Tips

Draw your tailbone down and under to counteract any excessive arch in the lower back. Breathe deeply—try not to hold your breath.

OTHER HELPFUL STRETCHES

Wrist Stretch

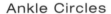

Helpful for: Carpal tunnel syndrome

Hold for 30 seconds

A. Flex your wrist so that your palm is facing forward and your fingers are pointing toward the ceiling. Use your other hand to gently pull the finger tips toward your body.

B. Next, turn your arm so that your palm is facing upward. As you flex the wrist, use the opposite hand to pull your fingertips toward your body.

Note: Never stretch to the point of extreme pain, and stop if you feel increased numbness and tingling. Gently hold the stretch at a comfortable point.

Ankle Circles

Helpful for: Easing leg cramps and improving flexibility

Reps: 10 in each direction

A. Sitting on a chair with your legs hanging toward the floor, rotate each ankle in full circles. This soothes leg cramps by increasing blood flow to the calves.

Hip Hike

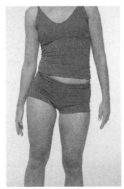

Helpful for: Easing round ligament pain

Reps: 8–10 on each leg

A. Stand tall with both knees slightly bent. Hike the right hip up, imagining that it is moving toward your bottom rib, then lower it back down. Complete 8–10 reps before moving to the other side.

Team Mallett Success Story

Laura Murton, 32, South Bloomfield, OH

Lost

19 pounds

4 dress sizes

24 total inches

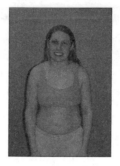
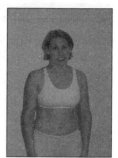

Before   After

• • • • •

Laura had always struggled with her body image, but this issue got worse during her pregnancy. "It was very difficult because I didn't like how I felt or looked," she recalls. Once her baby was born, she was determined to lose the 47 pounds that she had gained and feel good about her body. Having been a fan of Tracey's workout DVDs, Laura volunteered immediately when she heard that Tracey needed women to test drive the Super Fit Mama plan. "The thought of getting some personal help from Tracey was the additional motivation I needed," she recalls.

For a new mom like Laura, the quick Super Fit Mama workouts were ideal. "The fact that I could break them into smaller segments or do

---

TIPS FROM THE PROS: GOOD POSTURE DURING PREGNANCY

Heather Jeffcoat, DPT, Women's Physical Therapist

Follow these tips to help maintain good posture and ward off back pain during pregnancy:

1. Soften your knees so they remain unlocked and relaxed. Distribute your weight evenly toward the arches of your feet. These changes will also occur naturally as you tilt your pelvis back.
2. Pull your shoulder blades down and back to decrease rounding in your shoulders and upper back.
3. Tuck your chin so that your ears are over your shoulders.
4. Never wear high heels, as this accentuates the pregnant posture and will throw you further off balance.

This may feel awkward at first, but as you gain strength and flexibility, it will become second nature!

them all at once made exercising seem less daunting," she says. "It made it easier to stick with my workouts and not feel like a failure on the days when I only had energy to do a little bit." To Laura, the best part of the program was the snowball effect it had on her life. "All you have to do is put your mind to it and after the first few workouts you start to feel different and it feels good," she explains. "So you keep at it a bit more and before you know it you're eating better because you've been putting your hard work into your body. It's a wonderful cycle!"

Recently, she headed to work wearing jeans that she hadn't worn in six years. The irony? The last time she fit into those jeans she'd gotten to be that skinny in a very unhealthy way: taking diet pills with diet Mountain Dew and not eating. "Back then, I worked out twice a day for at least an hour and had a horrible self image!" she says. "Today, I'm so proud that I have lost these 13 pounds and 3 to 4 sizes, in a healthy manner!" Plus, adds Laura, "I also have more energy, a strong body, and a huge boost in my spirit and confidence. If that's not progress, I'm not sure what is!"

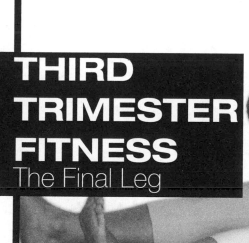

CHAPTER 4

THIRD TRIMESTER FITNESS
The Final Leg

THE MARATHON OF PREGNANCY CONTINUES, but the finish line—and your beautiful baby—are within sight. For me, the third trimester was the one in which I just couldn't seem to get comfortable. If you feel this way, too, it's with good reason. By now your baby has grown so much that your uterus almost fills your abdominal cavity (imagine that!) and this can press the diaphragm upward and make breathing more uncomfortable. If that's the case with you, it's probably time to turn down the intensity of your workouts. I'm not telling you not

YOUR BABY

- By 28 weeks your baby weighs as much as a Chinese cabbage.
- By 31 weeks your baby weighs as much as a large eggplant.
- By 33 weeks your baby weighs as much as a pineapple.
- By 36 weeks your baby weighs as much as a honeydew melon.
- By 39 weeks your baby weighs as much as a mini-watermelon.
- By 40 weeks your baby is about the size of a small pumpkin.

COMMON PHYSICAL CHANGES IN THE THIRD TRIMESTER

When I was pregnant, I felt like my body was an endless science experiment. I expected lots of changes in the first two trimesters but thought that by the third trimester things would slow down. No such luck. Here are a few things that you can expect in the last few months.

- Braxton Hicks are contractions that are said to be your body's way of practicing for the real thing. They tend to come and go unpredictably, and though they may catch you off guard, they're nothing to worry about. Contractions that lead to labor typically get longer, stronger, and closer together. Of course, if you're having contractions that concern you, contact your health-care provider.
- Breasts that keep on growing (and growing and growing!). Who knew that they could get any bigger, but they actually do. By now you have a whopping 1 to 3 extra pounds of breast tissue. As you get closer to your delivery date, don't be surprised if your nipples leak a yellowish fluid, which is called colostrum and is the milk that will feed your baby during his or her first few days of life.
- Stretch marks, unfortunately, don't need much explanation. These lovely pink, red, or purple streaks can appear on your stomach, breasts, butt, thighs, or arms. They're the result of the skin stretching, but whether or not you get them often has to do with genetics. Though experts say no cream can actually reduce stretch marks, some women find that moisturizing makes them less noticeable.
- Spider and varicose veins may begin to show up now. The boost in blood circulation in your body can lead to small reddish spots that sprout tiny blood vessels on your face, neck, upper chest, or arms, especially if you have fair skin. Varicose veins—blue or reddish lines beneath the surface of the skin—also may appear, particularly in the legs but also in the vulva. Elevating your feet and wearing support hose can help, but don't be surprised if these roadmaps on your body hang around well after your baby is born.
- Hemorrhoids are one of the not-so-pretty sides of pregnancy. These varicose veins that are in your rectum are the result of both the pressure of the baby and the straining that can occur due to pregnancy-induced

to exercise, but instead take breaks and give your body the extra TLC it needs right now.

The good news is that over the next three months, the baby will slowly drop down into your pelvis, which will make breathing easier. The bad news? You'll probably find yourself spending lots of time in the bathroom since your bladder is now compressed between the baby's head and your pubic bone! In my third trimester, I knew the location of every bathroom in town. But no story of mine compares to that of Jennifer, one of the women on Team Mallett. During her eighth month of pregnancy she went to the ladies' room and noticed that her underwear and jeans were soaked. She called her doctor, who told her to come into the hospital to see if her amniotic fluid was leaking. After two hours of waiting at the hospital and a rather horrific test, she called the whole family to tell them that she was not going into labor, but had unknowingly peed her pants!

(CONTINUED)

constipation. Try including plenty of fiber in your diet and drinking lots of fluids to get things moving down there.

- Edema is a fancy word for the swelling that occurs when you're a momma-in-the-making. This extra fluid is the result of a 50 percent increase in blood volume in the body. I had one friend whose hands blew up so much that they looked like they'd just been through a prize fight. Though this swelling of your hands, ankles, and feet can happen any time of day, it often occurs in the afternoon or evening, especially if you've been standing for a while. Try elevating your legs (gravity causes fluid to pool in your feet), wearing supportive shoes and pantyhose, steering clear of salty foods, and drinking at least eight 8-ounce glasses of water a day to help flush out your system. Natural diuretics like grapefruit and asparagus may also help. Just one important note: Mild puffiness is pretty common. However, if your hands and face become swollen or you have a sudden increase in swelling, see your doctor as soon as possible to rule out a serious medical condition like preeclampsia (pregnancy-induced hypertension), which can have dangerous complications. Headaches, changes in vision, nausea, dizziness, and decreased urine output are also signs of preeclampsia. Call your doctor immediately if you experience any of these symptoms.

- Heating up. If you're feeling the heat as this trimester progresses and find yourself sweating a lot, you're not alone. This is normal as your baby continues to grow. To stay cool, dress in breathable fabrics like cotton, avoid exercising outside in the middle of the day if temps are high, and steer clear of the sun. Cool off in a cold bath, shower, or pool or with a mini-fan by your side.

- Sleep doesn't come easily in this last trimester. Despite the fact that you may feel more exhausted and less energetic, it's often not that easy to catch your forty winks, because your huge stomach makes it hard to find a comfy position, you're frequently making midnight bathroom runs, and your body's metabolism can leave you sweating in your sheets. A few things that can help are avoiding large meals before bedtime, doing mild exercise like walking, and engaging in a relaxing activity before bedtime, like getting a rubdown from your mate, taking a warm bath, or reading a good book.

Another surprise during this trimester is how much *bigger* you'll get. I remember being in my seventh or eighth month and having a friend (a mother of three) tell me that *now* was when I'd get "really big." I took one look at my enormous stomach and rolled my eyes, thinking she was nuts, but she was right on. By the middle to end of my third trimester, I could barely see my feet. My belly got so huge (in addition to other body parts) that I was often asked if I was carrying twins!

Around this time, your nesting instinct may kick in and you can start to feel panicked if your nursery isn't ready or your house isn't baby-proofed. Just remember the baby has no clue (and couldn't care less) what the room looks like. Plus, he or she will probably sleep in your room for the first few months. Luckily the baby won't be moving around for a while, so you will have plenty of time to lock the cabinets and the toilet seat.

Lastly, if you're like me and flipping out because you're about to become a mom but have never changed a diaper, breastfed, or prepared a bottle, realize that you're not alone, which is why there are lots of baby-care and breastfeeding classes available. (Find one through your local hospital, OB/GYN, or pediatrician's office.) I actually found them very practical and they helped ease my anxiety.

THIRD TRIMESTER WORKOUT PLAN

The workout plan for this trimester contains some of the same exercises that are in the second trimester workout. However, some have been modified to take into consideration the impact your growing belly is having on your balance and ease of movement. Remember, you're now carrying more weight, so moving your body will require more energy at a time when you feel like you have none. Don't be hard on yourself. Just do what you can even if it's at a slower pace. Depending on how you feel

SIGNS OF LABOR

- Contractions at regular and increasingly shorter intervals that also become stronger in intensity.
- Lower back pain that doesn't go away. You might also feel premenstrual and crampy.
- Your water breaks. This can be a large gush or a continuous trickle.
- A bloody (brownish or blood-tinged) mucous discharge from the "mucous plug" that blocks the cervix

and how much weight you have gained, you can continue with the second trimester exercises and slowly start incorporating the third trimester variations.

To prepare you for labor I've added some super stretching exercises that will open the hips and keep this area flexible so you will be ready for the descent of the baby. Try and incorporate these relaxing and de-stressing stretches into your day most days of the week.

THIRD TRIMESTER CARDIO STRENGTH TRAINING CIRCUIT

Time: 6 to 8 minutes per circuit segment, not including the warm-up.

How to: Perform each exercise once using the recommended set of weights. Repeat if you'd like to do another set. I've suggested a number of reps for each exercise, but if you are just starting out, you may start lower and work up to these targets.

You'll need: Two sets of dumbbells, a chair, and a pillow. (Again, for each exercise I've indicated which set of dumbbells to use with the terms "Lighter" and "Heavier." These could be 3-lb. and 5-lb. weights, or, if you're just starting out, you might choose to use 1-lb. and 3-lb. weights instead, or 2-lb. and 4-lb. weights. If one set seems too heavy for you, go with a lighter set until you are ready to move up.)

CIRCUIT A

Warm-up: March in place for 1 or 2 minutes, making large, slow, rhythmic movements. Circle your arms forward and back while taking deep breaths.

1. Tricep stationary lunges

Muscles targeted: Quads, hamstrings, glutes, and triceps

Reps: 15 on each leg

Weights: Lighter

Tracey's Tips

Keep your knee over the first and second toe and make sure that your body is tall with the abs contracted. Gently hold the chair for support so that the hand is just resting on the top of it without any stress in the neck and shoulders.

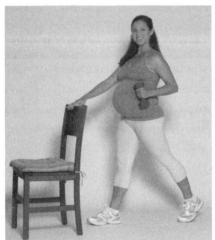

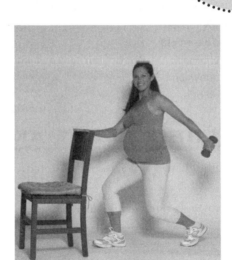

A. Start facing the chair with your right leg in front and left leg behind you. Make sure both feet are facing forward, with the back foot resting on a toe and your left arm bent with the elbow slightly behind your body.

B. Exhale, bend both knees into a lunge position, and extend your elbow as you contract the back of the upper arm (triceps). Inhale, straighten the knees, and bend the elbow back to start position.

2. Attitude side lift with shoulder raise, modified

Muscles targeted: Quads, glutes, and shoulders

Reps: 12 on each leg

Weights: Lighter

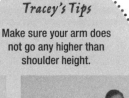

Tracey's Tips

Make sure your arm does not go any higher than shoulder height.

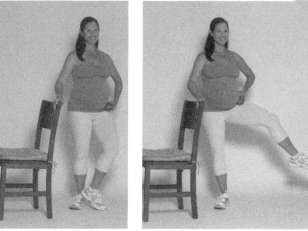

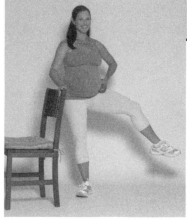

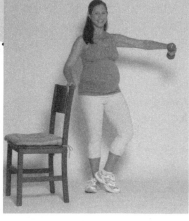

A. Stand beside the chair with your legs turned out at the hips and your outside (right) leg resting on a toe. Place your outside arm on your hip and the other hand on top of the chair.

Note: Place weights on the floor.

B. Lift your right leg off the floor with the knee slightly bent, but without hiking the hip. Your aim is to keep the hips level.

C. As you lower the leg back to the starting position, lift the outside arm out to the side to shoulder height, leading with the elbow.

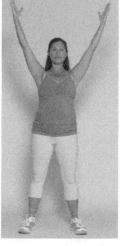

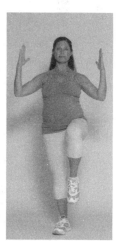

Cardio:

Knee raises for 60 seconds.

Start with your feet shoulder-width apart and your arms extended over your head. Exhale and bend your right knee toward the chest and the elbows down to the hips, then extend your arms back over your head and lower the right leg. Repeat on the other side. Alternate legs for 60 seconds.

3. Plié and pelvic tilt with "V" to "W" arms

Muscles targeted: Quads, hamstrings, abs, pelvic floor, and mid to upper back

Reps: 20

Weights: Lighter

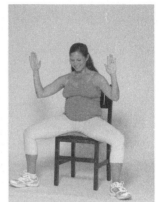

A. Start by sitting on the edge of a chair with your legs bent, open wide to the side of the body and turned out at the hips, and toes pointing out to the corners of the room. Place your arms over your head in a wide "V" position, pulling your shoulder blades down toward your pelvis.

B. Exhale and tilt your pelvis forward by contracting your abdominals and drawing your pubic bone up toward your belly button. At the same time, draw your elbows down toward your hips by contracting the lats (sides of the back). Then move the pelvis back to neutral (start position), extending the arms back to a "V" position. Repeat 20 times before extending the legs.

Tracey's Tips

Draw the pelvis slightly underneath you so as not to overarch the back. Keep the knees over the toes and the weight into your heels.

4. Squat row

Muscles targeted: Quads, hamstrings, glutes, and mid to upper back

Reps: 15

Weights: Heavier

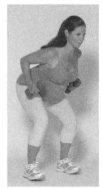

A. Start with your feet shoulder-width apart and your hands by the sides of your body. Rest your weight in your heels.

B. Go into a squat by bending your knees and reaching your arms forward. Exhale and squeeze your shoulder blades together, drawing your elbows back into a rowing position. Inhale and straighten your arms then knees. Repeat from the beginning for a total of 15 reps.

Note: Place weights on the floor.

Cardio:

Repeat knee raises for 60 seconds.

Cooldown: Walk or march in place for a few minutes to bring your heart rate down before moving on to the next circuit.

CIRCUIT B

1. Pliés with angle bicep curls

Muscles targeted: Quads, hamstrings, glutes, biceps, and shoulders

Reps: 12 on each side

Weights: Lighter

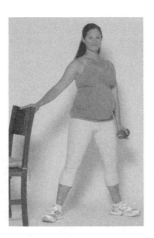 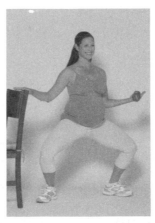

A. Start standing beside a chair with your feet shoulder-width apart, turned out at the hips with the toes pointing out to the corners of the room. Position your arms so that the outside arm is slightly bent, with the palm facing upward at hip height, and your inside arm is holding onto the chair for support. Bend both legs so that your knees are over your toes, and at the same time lift your outside arm up to shoulder height, then straighten your knees as you lower the arm back down.

B. Next, bend your knees, but this time bend the elbow into a bicep curl. Alternate arm lift with bicep curl for a total of 12 reps, then repeat by turning to the other side.

2. Squat with single arm posterior deltoid flies

Muscles targeted: Quads, hamstrings, glutes, and posterior deltoids

Reps: 12 on each side

Weights: Lighter

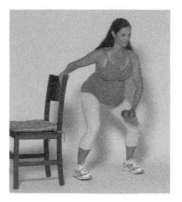

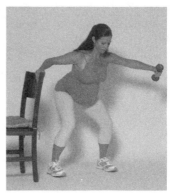

Tracey's Tips

Always draw in your abs and pull your shoulders down toward the pelvis. Keep your weight over your heels and your knees pointing forward.

A. Start beside the chair with your feet shoulder-width apart, toes pointing forward, and the right hand holding onto the chair for support. The left arm is slightly rounded in front of the body with the palm facing inward and your body slightly pitched forward from the waist.

B. Bend your knees as you shift your weight back into the heels and lift your left arm out to the side, leading with the elbow and drawing your left shoulder blade toward the middle of your back, then lower your arm as you straighten your legs. Do 12 reps before repeating on the other side.

Note: Place weights on the floor.

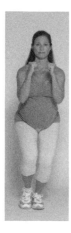

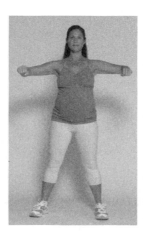

Cardio:

Traveling sideways squats for 60 seconds.

Take one step out to the side into a squat and then repeat in the same direction as you open the arms out to the side at shoulder height, leading with the elbows. Then go to the left for two traveling side squats.

3. Tricep dips

Muscles targeted: Triceps

Reps: 10–15

Weights: None

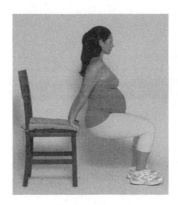

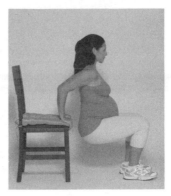

Note: This exercise is not appropriate for women suffering from carpal tunnel syndrome. If you have carpal tunnel problems, do the following standing triceps extension using light dumbbells instead of the chair version.

A. Start by sitting on the edge of a chair with your elbows bent, hands resting on the corners of the seat with fingers facing forward, knees bent hip-width apart, and spine in a neutral position.

B. Lift your hips off the seat and inhale as you bend your elbows, then exhale as you straighten your arms. Do 10–15 reps and then return to a sitting position.

Modification: Standing triceps extension

Muscles targeted: Triceps

Reps: 15–20

Weights: Lighter

A. Start with your legs hip-width apart, knees slightly bent, and your body slightly pitched forward from your hips. Bend the elbows so that they are positioned slightly behind your body.

B. Straighten the elbows, keeping the upper arms still and contracting the triceps (top of the back of the arms), as you fully extend the arms in a slow and controlled movement.

Tracey's Tips

Keep your shoulder blades down to decrease stress on the neck.

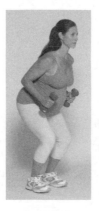

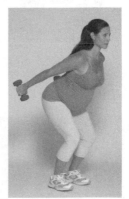

4. Lateral side leg lift with shoulders and biceps

Muscles targeted: Shoulders, biceps, and glutes

Reps: 12 on each leg

Weights: Lighter

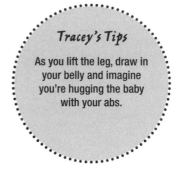

Tracey's Tips

As you lift the leg, draw in your belly and imagine you're hugging the baby with your abs.

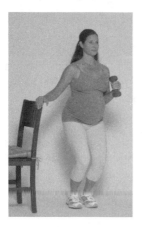 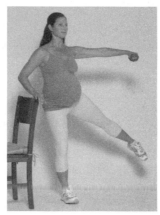

A. Start beside the chair with your legs together and your knees bent in a squat position, your left (outside) elbow bent, and your palm facing toward your body in a hammer bicep curl. The inside hand is resting on the chair for support. Extend the legs and rest the weight on the outside hip.

B. Exhale and lift the left (outside) leg out to the side of the body off the floor just below hip height. Make sure your toe is facing forward. Then lower the leg back into start position and repeat for 12 reps, then repeat on the other leg.

Modification: If this exercise is uncomfortable for you, don't lift the leg but simply extend it to a point on the floor.

Note: Place weights on the floor.

Cardio:

Repeat traveling sideways squats for 60 seconds.

Cooldown: Walk or march in place for a few minutes to bring your heart rate down before moving on to the next circuit.

CIRCUIT C

Note: No weights are needed for this workout.

1. Pliés

Muscles targeted: Glutes, hamstrings, quads, and abs for balance

Reps: 15–20

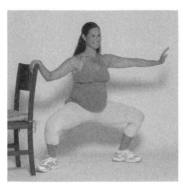

A. Start with your legs a little further than shoulder-width apart with your toes pointing to the corners of the room and your legs turned out at the hips. Your right arm is resting on the chair for support and your left arm is extended out to the side at shoulder height with the hand flexed.

B. Bend both knees into a plié position. Hold this plié while performing little up and down pulses, alternating lifting your heels off the floor for a total of 15–20 reps, then extend both legs.

Modifications: Do only pliés without lifting the heels off the floor if the heel rise is too difficult for you.

2. Arm circles

Muscles targeted: Shoulders, upper back, quads, hamstrings, and glutes

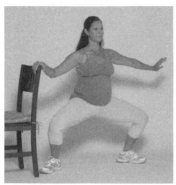

Reps: 15 slow circles forward and backward

A. Stand with your legs a little further than shoulder-width apart, toes pointing to the corners of the room and legs turned out at the hips. Your right arm is resting on the chair for support and your left arm is extended out to the side at shoulder height with the hand flexed.

B. Bend both knees into a plié position, circle the arm forward in small circles for 15 reps, then repeat in the opposite direction. Switch sides and repeat the sequence with the right arm.

Cardio:

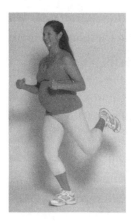

Hamstring curl for 60 seconds.

Step to the left, then bend the right knee, bringing the heel toward the butt, and bend your elbows at the side of your body. Repeat, alternating the legs for 60 seconds. Keep both knees bent at all times and focus on squeezing the hamstrings as you bring the heel to the butt.

3. Yoga chair

Muscles targeted: Glutes, hamstrings, quads, and calves

Reps: 20

Tracey's Tips

Press the weight into your heels during the squat and extend the upper spine, lifting the chest toward the ceiling.

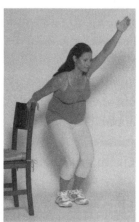

A. Start with your feet hip-width apart and your right arm holding onto a chair for support. Bend both knees into a squat, shifting your weight into your heels, and then lift your outside arm overhead in line with your ears, palms facing toward the body.

B. Curl the pelvis under, taking the arch out of the lower back. Then extend your legs and bring your body back to an erect position. Perform 20 reps.

4. Hitch a ride

Muscles targeted: Mid to upper back, shoulders, glutes, quads, and hamstrings

Reps: 15, with 20 pulses

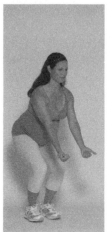 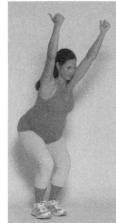

A. Start with your feet hip-width apart and knees bent with your weight in your heels. Your arms are straight in front of the body with your palms facing upward and your thumbs extended.

B. Exhale and lift your arms into a "V" position, leading with the thumbs, as you extend the spine, then bring your arms back to the start position. Do 15 reps, staying in a squat position, then perform 20 tiny up and down pulses.

Cardio:

Hamstring curl for 60 seconds.

Cooldown: Walk or march in place for a few minutes to bring the heart rate down gradually, taking nice deep breaths.

Tracey's Tips

As you lift your arms over your head, try to keep the shoulder blades drawing down and back so that you don't create stress in the neck and shoulders.

SUPER FIT MAMA CORE STRENGTHENING

Time: 6–8 minutes.

How to: Perform one set of each of the following exercises.

You'll need: Three pillows and a rolled-up towel.

Note: An asterisk (*) denotes that a core-strengthening exercise is safe to perform with diastasis recti.

1. Hip circles on all fours*

Muscles targeted: Abdominal and pelvic floor

Reps: 5 circles to the right and left

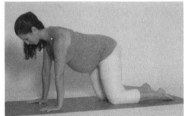

A. Position yourself on your hands and knees with your hands directly under your shoulders and your knees directly under your hips. Pull your abs in and keep your spine in a neutral position.

B. Inhale as you move your hips to the right and start to make a circle with the hips in a clockwise direction. As you exhale, draw in your abdominals. Pull up the pelvic floor as you finish the circle. Repeat 5 times then proceed to the other side.

Tracey's Tips

Keep your weight forward over your upper body and keep your shoulders over your hands. Focus on deep breathing to contract the abs and pelvic floor.

YOUR BODY

- You may experience achiness in your lower abdomen.
- You may see a heavy white discharge.
- You may experience an increase in heartburn, flatulence, bloating, and constipation or hemorrhoids.
- You may feel fatigued and have a difficult time sleeping.
- You may still be gaining an average of 1–2 pounds per week.

2. Wag the tail version 1*

Muscles targeted: Abdominals and pelvic floor

Reps: 8 to each side

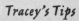

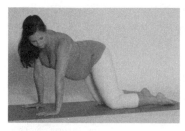

A. Position yourself on your hands and knees. Make sure your hands are shoulder-width apart and directly under your shoulders and your knees are stacked under your hips.

Tracey's Tips

As you do the pelvic tilt, contract the pelvic floor. Keep the stress out of your upper body by pulling your shoulders away from your ears and not sinking in between the shoulder blades.

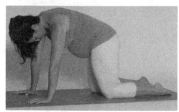

B. Move your hips to the right side as if you were a dog wagging your tail, then draw your abs in and do a pelvic tilt. Release the tilt then return to center and repeat to the other side.

3. Clams*

Muscles targeted: Abdominals, pelvic floor, and glutes

Reps: 15 on each side

Tracey's Tips

Keep your hips stacked and facing forward as you lift the knee. Imagine that your thigh bone is drawing in and up as your thigh moves up. Lift your knee only as high as you can without rotating the pelvis and lower spine. This is a great time to add Kegels, throughout the movement.

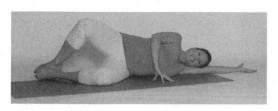

A. Start by lying on your right side with your knees bent, hips and knees stacked on top of each other. Extend your right arm on the floor and rest your right ear on the bicep. Place your left hand on your left hip.

B. Exhale and lift the top (left) knee toward the ceiling, keeping the heels together and the hips stacked. Inhale, lower the knee, and then repeat to the other side.

4. Cat pillow squeeze*

Muscles targeted: Inner thighs and pelvic floor

Reps: 15

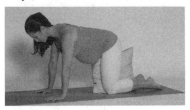

A. Position yourself on your hands and knees, with legs hip-width apart and a pillow between your inner thighs. Make sure your shoulders are over your hands and your hips are over your knees.

B. Squeeze the pillow and tilt your pelvis, drawing your abdominals in toward the spine and your pubic bone toward the belly button, and pull up the pelvic floor like an elevator. Inhale and return to the neutral position. Repeat 15 times.

Tracey's Tips

Imagine that you're drawing your knees together and focus on the inner thighs doing all the work. Be sure to contract the pelvic floor.

Focus on drawing in your abdominals at all times and contracting the pelvic floor on every exhale.

5. Knee lifts walking in place*

Muscles targeted: Abdominals and pelvic floor

Reps: 10 on each side

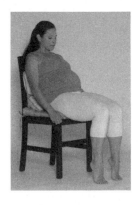
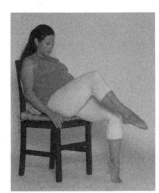

A. Place a pillow at a diagonal resting on the back of the chair. Sit down with your tailbone a few inches from the end of the chair and your upper body against the back so that your body is on an incline. Bend your knees, with the balls of your feet resting on the floor and your toes pointing forward.

B. Exhale and lift the right leg off the floor toward your chest, then inhale and lower your leg back to the start position. Alternate your legs as you "walk in place" for 10 reps on each leg.

6. Plank forearm on knees

Muscles targeted: Abdominals

Hold for 20–30 seconds

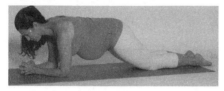

A. Begin in a modified plank position, face down and body diagonal to the floor, balancing on your forearms with your elbows bent, knees bent and resting on the floor. Your shoulders are directly in line with your elbows, and your body is a diagonal from the crown of the head to your knees. Hold this position for 20–30 seconds by drawing in your abdominals and pressing the pelvis forward.

Tracey's Tips

Be careful not to overarch your back. Focus on the exhale as you pull the belly in and the pelvic floor up. Imagine you're in a slight pelvic tilt and drawing the pelvic floor up.

7. T-stand*

Muscles targeted: Total body

Hold for 30 seconds

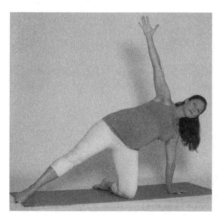

A. Start by sitting on your right hip with your knees bent and your right elbow bent, your forearm resting on the floor with your fingers pointing forward. Your left arm is by your left hip.

B. Exhale and lift the hips off the floor, extend the left leg straight out to the side, and reach the left arm up at shoulder height, palms facing outward. Hold for 30 seconds. Lower your hips as you bend your left knee and bring your arm back to the side of the body. Repeat on the other side.

Tracey's Tips

Keep the shoulder blades pulling down toward the hips, especially on the supporting arm, to avoid tension in the shoulder and neck. Avoid overarching the back by keeping the abs contracted at all times.

8. Spine stretch with thumb pulses*

Muscles targeted: Mid to upper back and hamstrings

Reps: 8 with 8 pulses each

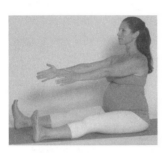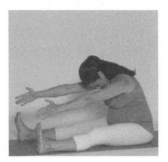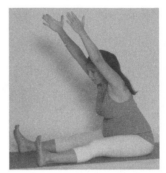

A. Sitting tall on the floor or on a pillow (the pillow is especially good if you have tight hamstrings), extend your legs in front of you shoulder-width apart, and extend your arms out in front of you at shoulder height.

B. Exhale, contract the abs, and curl up and over, as if you're going up and over a big beach ball as you reach forward toward your feet.

C. Inhale and extend the spine as you move your arms so that your biceps are by your ears. With thumbs on top, gently pulse the thumbs up to the ceiling as you draw your shoulder blades down the back to work on the mid to upper back. Exhale and curl forward, up over your beach ball, to return to the start position

Tracey's Tips

Imagine that you have a beach ball sitting in front of your torso as you reach up and over toward the feet, drawing in the abdominals tight.

SUPER FIT MAMA FLEXIBILITY AND HIP OPENER SEGMENT

Time: About 6 minutes (if you feel like holding the stretches for longer than the designated times, go ahead. You deserve a little pampering— you have earned it!).

How to: Try to perform these stretches on most days of the week. They will help to ease discomfort as you're nearing the end of your pregnancy.

You'll need: A chair and a pillow.

1. Sitting glute stretch

Muscles targeted: Glutes and the piriformis

Hold for 30 seconds on each side

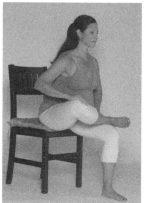

A. Sitting tall toward the edge of a chair, bend the right leg and turn out at the hip. Flex your right foot and rest your ankle on top of your left thigh. Place your right arm onto your right knee and your left hand onto your left knee.

B. Hinge forward from your hips to the point where you feel a comfortable stretch in your glutes. Then repeat with the other leg.

Tracey's Tips

To open your hip a little bit more, add gentle resistance on your bent leg. Take deep breaths during the stretches, slowly inhaling and exhaling.

Focus on pressing the pelvis forward in a tilt and hugging the baby with your abs. You will feel a greater stretch in the hip and thigh and less strain in the lower back.

2. Sitting hip flexor stretch

Muscles targeted: Hip flexors and quads

Hold for 30 seconds on each leg

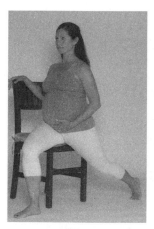

A. Sitting on the edge of the chair with your legs open a little further than shoulder-width apart, turn your pelvis to the right side so that your hips are facing to the right.

B. Bend your right knee and extend the left leg behind you, then press the hips forward, pulling the abs in toward the spine. You will feel a stretch through the front of the thigh. Reach your arms over your head with your palms facing toward each other. Hold for 30 seconds and then repeat on the other side.

Modification: If balance becomes an issue, place one hand on the chair for support and the other on the hip.

3. Sitting hamstring stretch

Muscles targeted: Hamstrings

Hold for 30 seconds on each leg

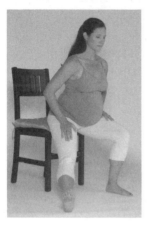

A. Sit tall on the edge of the chair, bend your right leg, and extend your left leg slightly out on a diagonal, resting on a heel, to make room for your belly.

B. Hinge forward from your hips, extending the upper spine and leading with the sternum. Repeat on the other side.

Tracey's Tips

Keep your hips facing forward and breathe while holding the stretch.

If this exercise feels uncomfortable, place two pillows under each knee for extra support.

4. Butterfly

Muscles targeted: Inner thighs

Hold for 30 seconds

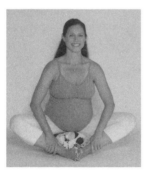

A. Sit down on the floor or on a pillow and place the soles of your feet together with your knees wide and out to the sides. Hold onto your shins and place your elbows on top of the inner thighs to create gentle resistance, then open the hips a little further.

B. Leading with the sternum, hinge your torso forward from the hips and hold, gently trying to increase the stretch in the hips.

EXERCISE POINTERS

1. As mentioned earlier, during squats and pliés you can add a Kegel—a great way to get in your recommended daily amount.
2. If you have carpel tunnel syndrome, keep your wrists neutral rather than bending them; if pain persists, try a lower weight or no weight.

5. Mermaid in Z position with QL stretch

Muscles targeted: Obliques, lower back, and quadratus lumborum

Hold for 30 seconds in each position

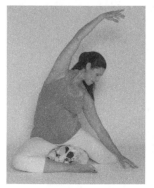 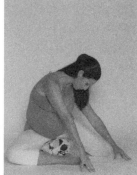

A. Sitting on your right hip with your right leg bent forward and your left leg bent toward the back in a Z position, place your right hand on the floor and your left hand overhead in a side stretch.

B. Hold the stretch and take deep breaths, then reach diagonally forward and curve your upper body forward. Hold again and breathe deeply, then lift back up to center. Repeat on the other side.

6. Birthing squat

Muscles targeted: Quads, hamstrings, glutes, and pelvic floor

Hold for 30 seconds

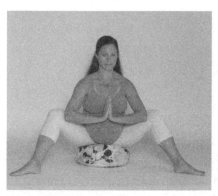

A. Sit on the edge of a chair with your legs shoulder-width apart. Your toes are pointing to the corners of the room and your legs are turned out at the hips. Shift your weight into your heels and place your hands together in a prayer position in front of the chest. Hold this position for 30 seconds.

Modification: Sit tall on the edge of a chair with your legs bent and turned out at the hips.

7. Standing tree pose

Muscles targeted: Legs, glutes, and abs

Hold for 15–30 seconds

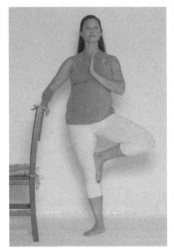

A. Start by standing tall beside a chair, holding onto the chair with your left hand. Place the right hand in a prayer position. Turn the right leg out at the hip, bend the right knee, and rest the right foot just above the left knee. Draw in your abs, balance, and hold the pose, then switch to the other side.

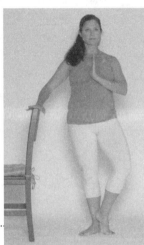

Modification: If this proves to be too challenging for your sense of balance, balance on the ball of your foot instead of lifting the leg or don't lift the leg as high, and position the hand facing toward your heart.

Tracey's Tips

Focus on an object at eye level to help you balance.

Take the strain out of the shoulders by pulling the shoulder blades down the back and gently hold onto the chair without tension. Draw in the abdominals so that the back does not overarch.

8. Table top

Muscles targeted: Upper and lower back and hamstrings

Hold for 30 seconds

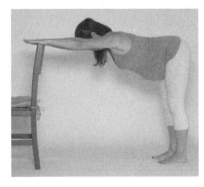

A. Stand behind the chair with your hands on its back corners, walk back a few steps, and bend at the hips, keeping a flat back.

B. Keep your legs straight and your feet, knees, and hips in one straight line. Your toes are pointing forward. Hold for 30 seconds, taking deep breaths and focusing on opening the upper back, and drawing the abs in to support the lower back.

CIRCUIT A

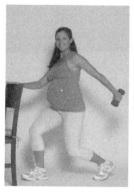 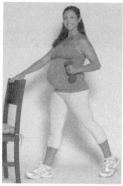

1. TRICEP STATIONARY LUNGES

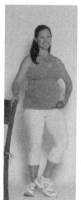 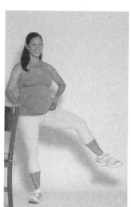 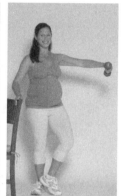

2. ATTITUDE SIDE LIFT WITH SHOULDER RAISE, MODIFIED

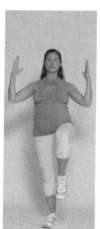

CARDIO: KNEE RAISES FOR 60 SECONDS

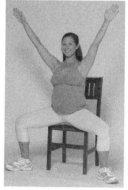

3. PLIÉ AND PELVIC TILT WITH "V" TO "W" ARMS

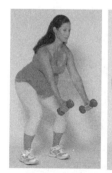

4. SQUAT ROW

CARDIO: REPEAT KNEE RAISES FOR 60 SECONDS

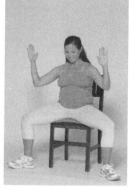

CIRCUIT B

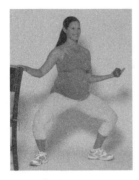
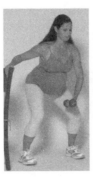
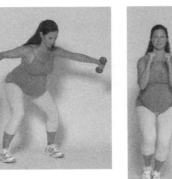
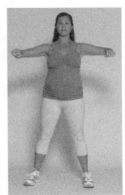

1. PLIÉS WITH ANGLE BICEP CURLS

2. SQUAT WITH SINGLE ARM POSTERIOR DELTOID FLIES

CARDIO: TRAVELING SIDEWAYS SQUATS FOR 60 SECONDS.

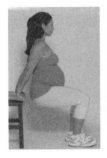
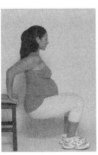
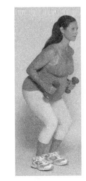

3. TRICEP DIPS

MODIFICATION: STANDING TRICEPS EXTENSION

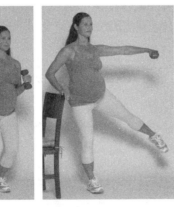

4. LATERAL SIDE LEG LIFT WITH SHOULDERS AND BICEPS

CARDIO: REPEAT TRAVELING SIDEWAYS SQUATS FOR 60 SECONDS.

CIRCUIT C

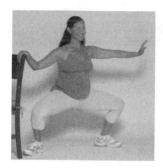

1. PLIÉS

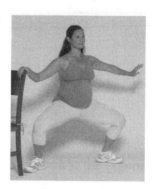

2. ARM CIRCLES

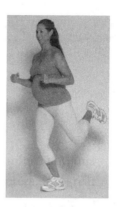

CARDIO: HAMSTRING CURL FOR 60 SECONDS.

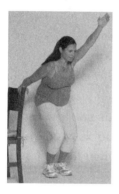

3. YOGA CHAIR

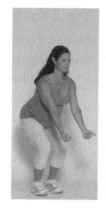

4. HITCH A RIDE

CARDIO: REPEAT HAMSTRING CURL FOR 60 SECONDS.

CORE STRENGTHENING

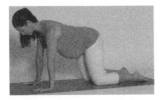

1. HIP CIRCLES ON ALL FOURS*

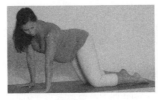
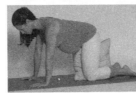

2. WAG THE TAIL VERSION 1*

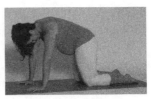

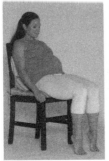

3. CLAMS*

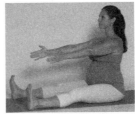

4. CAT PILLOW SQUEEZE*

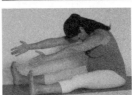

6. PLANK FOREARM ON KNEES

5. KNEE LIFTS WALKING IN PLACE*

8. SPINE STRETCH WITH THUMB PULSES*

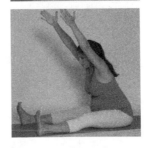

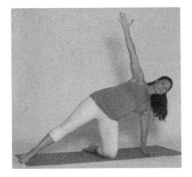

7. T-STAND*

SUPER FIT MAMA FLEXIBILITY AND HIP OPENER SEGMENT

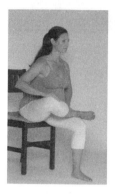 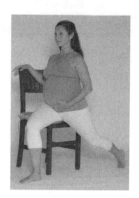 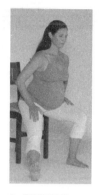 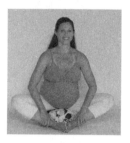

1. SITTING GLUTE STRETCH

2. SITTING HIP FLEXOR STRETCH

3. SITTING HAMSTRING STRETCH

4. BUTTERFLY

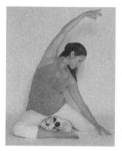 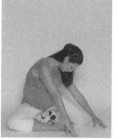

5. MERMAID IN Z POSITION WITH QL STRETCH

6. BIRTHING SQUAT

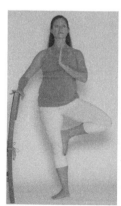 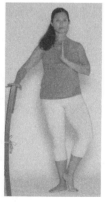

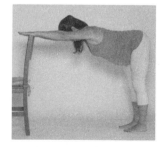

7. STANDING TREE POSE

8. TABLE TOP

PARTNER STRETCHES

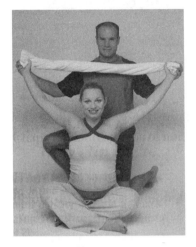

1. CHEST OPENER

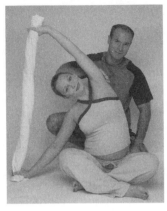

2. SIDE STRETCH

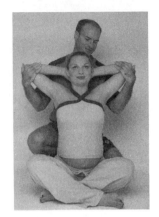

3. CHEST STRETCH

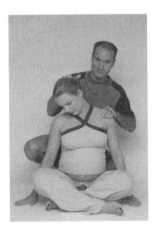

**4. NECK AND UPPER
BACK STRETCH**

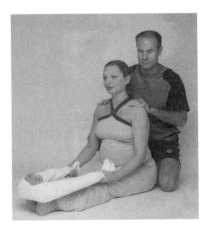

5. HAMSTRING STRETCH

PARTNER STRETCHES

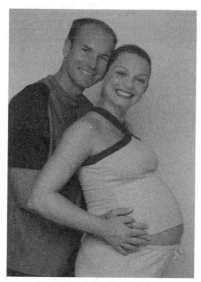

Tracey 8 months pregnant and husband, Dr. Chris Mallett.

Not only do these exercises prepare you for the delivery room, but they'll ward off pain by allowing your muscles to be flexible and strong even when the extra weight of your baby starts pulling on your lax ligaments and joints. Adding a partner to your stretches provides extra resistance. (However, you can perform these exercises solo simply by using a towel.)

Another reason I love these partner stretches is that they're a good way for you and your mate to connect, something that's important since your daddy-to-be often feels a little left out. These exercises are helpful beyond pregnancy, too. In fact, I still do most of them daily to help improve my posture and prevent any more shoulder injuries.

The following four exercises are designed to help correct the poor posture and tight chest muscles that can accompany pregnancy. This happens when your belly's extra weight causes the lower spine to arch and the upper spine to round forward. And trust me, at this point of your pregnancy you will want to do these exercises because they feel oh-so-good!

Time: About 6 minutes.

How to: Hold each stretch for at least 30–60 seconds for maximum benefit.

You'll need: A rolled-up towel or exercise band, a pillow, and a chair.

1. Chest opener

Purpose: This exercise stretches out tight shoulders and opens the chest. Inspiration: Better posture and prevention of shoulder, neck, and upper back injuries.

Reps: 8–10

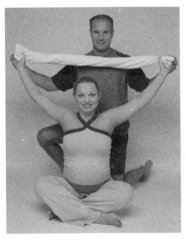

A. Sit crossed-legged on the floor or on a pillow or chair, depending on whatever feels the most comfortable. Holding a rolled-up towel, extend your arms in front of your chest and pull your hands away from each other so that the towel is taut.

B. Exhale and take your arms overhead and past your ears (still holding the towel) until you feel the stretch in your chest and shoulders.

C. Have your partner stand behind you and gently pull your arms to add a little resistance and increase the stretch. Hold this position for four breath cycles, then bring your arms back to the start position on an exhale.

2. Side stretch

Purpose: This one stretches the sides of the waist, the obliques and the lats, enabling them to function more freely. It really soothed the lower back pain that I experienced.

Hold for 30–60 seconds.

A. Start in the same position as in the chest opener with the towel in your hands overhead.

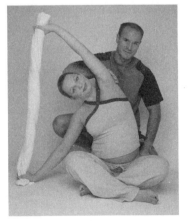

B. Exhale, reaching over to the right side and placing your hand closest to the floor on the mat. Keeping the towel taut, pull your hands away from each other, increasing the stretch in the side of the torso.

C. Have your partner place his right hand on your upper rib cage and his left hand on your left hip. Gently elongate the muscles and open this area by imagining that you're moving your hands away from each other. Hold this position for four breath cycles. Return to the starting position on an exhale, focusing on the obliques to bring you back to an erect position, then repeat to the other side.

3. Chest stretch

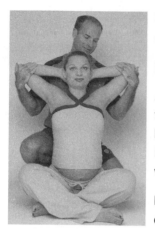

Purpose: This stretch is for the chest and shoulders.

Hold for 30–60 seconds.

A. Start by sitting cross-legged on the floor or pillow with your elbows bent and hands behind your head. Extend your upper spine, leading upward with the sternum.

B. Have your partner sit behind you and gently hold onto your elbows, creating an extra stretch.

Tracey's Tips

Draw your abs toward the spine to help prevent overarching of the back. This also helps you feel the stretch more in your chest rather than your lower back.

4. Neck and upper back stretch

Purpose: This stretch will help soothe tight neck muscles from the natural forward position of the head that often occurs in pregnancy.

Hold for 30 seconds.

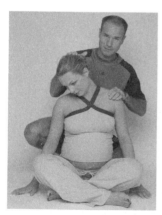

A. Start by sitting on the floor or a pillow with your legs crossed, or sitting tall on a chair. Place your right hand on your head and gently pull it to the side, stretching out the left side of the neck. Have your partner stand behind you with one hand on your left shoulder and the other on top of your right hand. Imagine you're pulling the hands apart to encourage a greater stretch.

B. Turn your head toward the right so that you are looking toward your right shoulder. Have your partner hold your left shoulder down so that it doesn't lift up and place his other hand on top of yours to gently increase the stretch. You will feel this stretch in the mid to upper back.

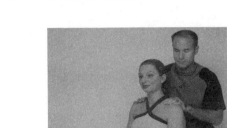

5. Hamstring stretch

Purpose: The following stretch will help with tight hamstrings, which can place a strain on the lower back. By keeping your hamstrings flexible, you can help to prevent or alleviate back and sciatica pain. Keeping the pelvis flexible is also crucial at this time as your body gets ready for labor and delivery.

Hold for 30 seconds on each leg.

A. Start by sitting down on the floor or on a pillow with your legs extended in front of you. Wrap a rolled-up towel around the arches of your feet and hold onto the ends of the towel.

B. Extend the body forward as if you were hinging from the hips. Lead with the sternum.

C. Have your partner sit behind you, gently placing a hand on your mid-back and slightly pushing forward to increase the stretch.

Team Mallett Success Story

Nicole Pascoe, 37, Wales, Great Britain

Lost

18 pounds

2 dress sizes

13 total inches

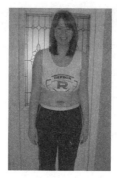 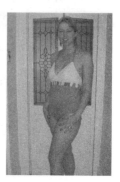

Before   After

• • • • •

Embarrassed by her body, Nicole, a mother of three, only took her children swimming when they were on vacation and nobody at the pool knew her. "My husband took them to our local pool or swimming parties while I sat inside and watched from the window." Nicole was unhappy about this, but she wasn't the only one. "My six-year-old son told my husband that it made him sad that I sat alone when they were having fun," she recalls. "It made me feel awful."

That was before she joined Team Mallett. "For the first time, I concentrated on looking good and feeling fit rather than what size I would be," she recalls. Nicole learned to eat healthy foods and the right portion sizes. Just a few weeks into the program, she attended a birthday party at an all-you-can-eat buffet. "The strangest thing happened: While my friends were eating two or three platefuls, I only managed one, which is about half of what I used to eat at those things," she says. "I think both my stomach shrunk and I reprogrammed my brain. It was great not to feel bloated like I normally would the next day."

Eating isn't the only thing that got easier. "Exercise has genuinely become part of my life and I can't imagine *not* doing it. In fact, when I feel my stress levels soaring, I have to get my exercise fix, even if it's just a few minutes," says Nicole. "What I love about this plan is that I don't have to pay for an expensive gym membership or find babysitters." Even better than the money she's saved is the new body she's earned.

When she first started the plan, friends and colleagues weren't very supportive. "Even after six weeks, I got negative comments about how I was bound to put the weight back on or how I could never keep up this level of exercise with three kids," she recalls. "It was difficult, but deep down I knew this program was different and I felt really positive."

That attitude paid off, and now Nicole's naysayers are singing a different tune. "The best thing about this plan is the inches that I've lost off my tummy. To have a flat stomach after giving birth to three kids is just amazing," she exclaims. "Relatives say this is the slimmest they've seen me in years," she says. "For the first time ever, I didn't mind being videotaped," says Nicole, who has come a long way from that mom who used to sit inside while her kids played in the pool. "For a recent family vacation, I wore shorts and a tankini everyday and felt great!"

CHAPTER 5

EATING FOR TWO

A FRIEND ONCE SAID TO ME, "NEVER GET IN A PREGNANT woman's way when she's hungry." After two pregnancies I couldn't agree more! And I'm not alone. Some of my friends believe that food tasted so much better when they were pregnant, and many women agree.

Though you're *supposed* to be gaining weight during this time, many women are surprised to learn that you only need 100 extra calories a day in the first trimester and just 300 extra in the second and third trimesters. The latter is the equivalent of a small bowl of cereal with milk, two scrambled eggs with cheese, two slices of toast and an egg, or a bagel. (If you're having twins, that number increases to 500 more calories daily.) During my first pregnancy when I really packed on the pounds, it wasn't from eating tons of junk, but from consuming portions that were way too big (as well as a few too many pints of ice cream). And though you need to consume more calories, those calories should be nutritionally rich. Making sure that you're eating a balanced diet will guarantee that you take in all the vitamins and minerals that are essential for your health and that of your growing baby.

Don't be so afraid to gain weight that you restrict your diet. This is a big no-no because without adequate nutrition, you riok your baby's health and development.

Not only does your baby use the foods you eat to grow and develop properly, much research shows that what you eat while pregnant can impact your child's weight and risk of diseases like diabetes and heart disease well into childhood and young adulthood. I truly believe that pregnancy is the perfect time to turn over a new leaf in terms of living a healthier life, and this includes cleaning up your diet. After all, now you have another person who is relying on you completely—while you're

VEGETARIANS

Meeting all your protein needs during pregnancy or while breastfeeding isn't easy if you're a vegetarian, so if this is a concern to you, talk to your physician or consult with a dietician. Aim to include various sources of high-quality, non-animal protein in your diet such as legumes (black beans, soybeans, lentils, tofu, tempeh), whole grains, seeds, and nuts. If you're a lacto-ovo vegetarian, dairy foods like low-fat cheese, milk, yogurt, and eggs are other good options. Eat a protein-rich food with every meal, and take a supplement of vitamin B12, a nutrient typically found in meat that helps the baby grow new cells. For women who do not drink milk or get a lot of sun exposure, a vitamin D supplement is needed now as well as after pregnancy for healthy bones.

pregnant and for at least eighteen years postpartum—and if that's not motivation to get healthy, I don't know what is.

Gaining too much weight also increases your risk of things like gestational diabetes and high blood pressure, which is a symptom of preeclampsia. On top of that, a recent study from Cornell University found that packing on too many pounds can turn a nine-month weight gain into a permanent one. Researchers there looked at 540 women and found that one year postpartum half of the women weighed more than they did before they got pregnant, while a quarter were more than 10 pounds heavier.

With my second pregnancy, I discovered that one key way to handle cravings and maintain my energy was to eat like a cow. By that I *don't* mean eating huge portions of everything in sight, but instead grazing on little bits of food throughout the day. This not only prevents nausea, because your stomach is never totally empty, but also helps your body better absorb nutrients and wards off heartburn and indigestion—both of which are common in pregnancy because the digestive system tends to slow down.

NUTRIENT MUST-HAVES FOR MOMS-TO-BE AND NEW MOMS

Your overall pregnancy diet needs to be well-balanced to ensure that you and your baby receive the right vitamins and minerals. And your post-pregnancy diet needs to be healthy in order to help you heal, slim down, and produce enough milk with all the essential nutrients if you're breastfeeding.

Carbohydrates (Grains)

If you were going low-carb before you got pregnant, now's the time to welcome carbs back into your diet. Carbohydrates, which consist of fiber, starches, and sugars, provide energy for your baby to grow, something that's especially important during those last few months of pregnancy (which is why most of your extra calories should come from carbs at that time). They also give you the energy and stamina that you need to power through each day (during and after pregnancy) and fight fatigue and nausea.

The best sources are complex carbs because they keep your sugar levels consistent and thus maintain your energy level. Whole grains, brown rice, whole-wheat bread, beans, and fruits and veggies are perfect choices. Sugar, on the other hand, isn't the best choice. In fact, you should really limit the sweet treats, since they can contribute to gestational diabetes during pregnancy and make it hard to shed pounds after your baby is born. Post-pregnancy, fibrous foods are the key to weight loss because they fill you up (and keep you satisfied longer) and they're low in fat. This is one of the main reasons why the Super Fit Mama post-pregnancy food plan includes an unlimited amount of veggies.

For nutritious ideas about how to reduce nausea during the first trimester, see the sidebar in Chapter 2 entitled "Managing Morning Sickness."

Another reason why carbs are a must for both moms-to-be and new moms: They are a great way to keep your mood lifted and calm yourself when stressed. A study at Massachusetts Institute of Technology's Clinical Research Center found that following a low-carb diet decreased the brain's production of serotonin, a feel-good chemical that regulates your mood. But eating a small amount of carbs during times of stress will help to release this calming chemical.

EDIBLES TO AVOID

- **Alcohol.** It's unclear what, if any, amount of alcohol is safe during pregnancy. Research shows that it can increase your baby's risk of birth defects even during the earliest weeks after conception.
- **Fish that contains mercury.** The Food and Drug Administration (FDA) and the Environmental Protection Agency (EPA) suggest that pregnant women, nursing moms, and young children avoid fish and shellfish that are high in mercury. Mercury can harm a fetus's or young child's developing nervous system, the lungs, the kidneys, and vision and hearing. Don't eat shark, swordfish, king mackerel, or tilefish, and limit fish lower in mercury—such as shrimp, canned light tuna, salmon, and catfish—to 12 ounces per week.
- **Unpasteurized foods.** This includes milk and soft cheeses (like brie, feta, camembert, and blue cheese), which may contain listeria, a food-borne bacteria that can be harmful or even fatal to your baby or to you. This is because your immune system is suppressed while you are pregnant, so you're up to twenty times more likely to become infected than nonpregnant women. Though some women think it's okay to eat these foods once in a while, experts suggest avoiding them completely until after your baby is born.
- **Raw and undercooked meats and fish.** Raw or undercooked meats and fish (like sushi)—as well as precooked items like hot dogs and cold cuts—may contain a parasite called *toxoplasmosis*. Make sure all meats and fish are well-cooked. (Note: Toxoplasmosis may also be found in cat feces, so have someone else clean that litter box if you have a cat.)
- **Unwashed fruits and veggies.** Get rid of any dirt, contaminants, or pesticides on fruits and veggies by scrubbing them clean with water, or buy a special cleaner made for this purpose. One I like is Environne Veggie Wash (www.vegiwash.com).
- **Dietary and herbal supplements.** Some of these products may not be safe to take when you're pregnant, so check with your doctor or midwife before taking any supplements.

The carbs that you should kiss good-bye (or at least limit in your diet) are white bread, pasta, and white rice, as well as foods that contain refined flour (like cakes and cookies), refined sugar, and high-fructose corn syrup. Foods like these will sabotage your efforts to eat a balanced, clean diet. They're also high-glycemic foods, which is a fancy way of saying that they spike your sugar level, giving you a quick hit of energy only to cause you to crash soon afterward. That's when you find yourself looking for food (often high-fat, over-processed foods) to keep you going. Unfortunately, a lot of the food that's considered "kids' food" contains these unhealthy ingredients, so it's no wonder we have an obesity epidemic.

DID YOU KNOW?

Though most doctors say a little coffee or caffeinated soda is okay while pregnant, new research shows that you may want to rethink a second or third cup. A study reported in the *American Journal of Obstetrics and Gynecology* found that women who sipped just 200 milligrams of caffeine a day (that's the equivalent of two cups of regular coffee or five cans of soda) in the first twenty weeks of pregnancy had twice the risk of miscarrying compared to those who kicked their caffeine habit.

Fiber

Fiber is a wonder food when you're trying to slim down because it keeps you feeling fuller for longer periods of time. Try to eat at least 20–35 grams a day. Fiber, which is found in many foods, including grains, vegetables, and fruits, also helps ease pregnancy-induced constipation because it softens and adds bulk to your stools, enabling your intestines to pass them more quickly and easily. Alleviating constipation wards off hemorrhoids, another not-so-pretty side effect of pregnancy, since you're not straining. Just one word of advice: When you up your fiber intake, remember to also up your fluid intake to help keep things moving along.

Examples of healthy fiber options:
1 piece whole wheat bread (3 grams of fiber)
½ cup brown rice (2 grams of fiber)
¾ cup bran cereal (8 grams of fiber)
½ cup garbanzo beans (6 grams of fiber)
¼ cup sunflower seeds (3 grams of fiber)
Medium apple (3–4 grams of fiber)
Medium orange (2–3 grams of fiber)

Fruits and Veggies

If it's hard for you to get your fill of fruits and veggies, you're not alone. The number one complaint from Team Mallett was that there was never enough time in the day to consume four servings of produce. However, when I pointed out the fact that they used to find the time to eat four servings of cookies or ice cream, they realized that it's all about making the right choices.

But if it's been ages since a veggie has passed through your lips, don't worry. Pregnancy is the perfect time to start a healthy relationship with food and stop the yo-yo dieting many of us have tried in the past. And you don't have to memorize any nutritional content—instead aim to eat a rainbow of fruits and veggies in different colors every day, and you'll easily reap the benefits of an array of vitamins and minerals. Citrus fruits, broccoli, and tomatoes are good choices for Vitamin C, and dark leafy greens are a great way to get the Vitamin A, folate, and iron that you need during pregnancy and breastfeeding. Sweet potatoes and squash, high in fiber and vitamins A and C, make a great choice for a nutritious side dish or as ingredients in soups and casseroles. Here are a few good ideas to help you get your fill of fruits and veggies:

- Aim to eat a piece of fruit or a vegetable at each meal. Give yourself bonus points for eating both!
- Pre-wash and cut your produce and then place it at the front of a refrigerator shelf, ideally one that's at eye-level. This way you can easily grab a healthy snack when you're hungry. If you're on the

TRACEY'S TOP FIVE PREGNANCY FOOD TIPS

If you get nothing else out of this chapter, these five tips are key!

1. Add 100 calories a day to your diet in your first trimester and 300 in your second and third trimesters. If you're expecting twins, bump that number up to 500 calories.
2. Eat six to seven small meals a day (breakfast, mid-morning snack, lunch, mid-afternoon snack, dinner, and evening snack if needed), and never go more than three hours without eating.
3. Never skip breakfast, and never go on a fast, even for a day. Fasting can increase the risk of your body going into *ketosis*, a serious condition that increases the acidity of the blood and may cause preterm labor. This is also one of many reasons not to diet during pregnancy.
4. Take a prenatal vitamin every day, but don't rely solely on your vitamin pills for healthy nutrients. Food should always be your first source for nutrition.
5. Eat an abundance of fruits, veggies, whole grains, and calcium-rich foods throughout your pregnancy.

go, pack some fruits or veggies in plastic baggies or containers to take with you.

- Try to eat a dark green, leafy side salad with baby tomatoes and raw broccoli at lunch or dinner.
- View fruits and veggies as natural medicines that can heal and prevent illness, not only for you but for your children.

Protein

Since protein is one of the essential building blocks for muscle, tissue, and new cells, getting the required amount is crucial when you're pregnant and post-pregnancy when you're exercising and trying to build new muscle. Great sources are chicken, turkey, beef, lamb, veal, liver, ham, canned tuna, wild salmon, flounder, trout, and shrimp as well as dairy foods like milk, yogurt, soy milk, tofu, cheese, cottage cheese, and eggs. Eat a maximum of 6 ounces of tuna per week, opting for light tuna instead of albacore, to keep your mercury intake low. According to the Environmental Working Group (EWG) and *Science* magazine, it's best to limit your intake of farmed salmon to one serving a month due to the contamination of PCBs, the environmental toxic waste found mostly in the fatty part of the fish. The EWG released a statement reporting that farmed salmon purchased in the United States has sixteen times the PCBs found in wild salmon. Peanut butter, black beans, chickpeas, lentils, navy beans, pinto beans, peas, soybeans, and lima beans are also good protein options during pregnancy.

One of my favorite sources of protein is whey protein because it's quickly absorbed by the body and gives you antioxidant protection, too. The perfect way to add whey protein into your diet is through smoothies, which can be powerful fiber-, calcium-, and protein-rich drinks in the morning or post-workout. (Team Mallett found the smoothie recipes in Chapter 11 to be an integral part of their healthy eating plan, giving them energy during mid-afternoon slumps and keeping them from picking unhealthy choices in between meals.)

If possible, go organic. Research from the *British Journal of Nutrition* found that eating at least 90 percent organic dairy and meat products may result in breast milk with higher levels of conjugated linoleic acid (CLA), which experts believe may boost the baby's immune system and help ward off heart disease, cancer, and diabetes well into adulthood.

Another good protein source is soy—especially if you're a vegetarian—because it also contains isoflavones, a type of phytoestrogen that experts say may help prevent breast cancer, menopausal symptoms, heart disease, and osteoporosis. Today, it's easier than ever to find foods made of soy, such as tofu, tempeh, edamame, soy burgers, soy milk, and soy butter, among others. With all the delicious options, it's not hard to get your recommended daily intake of about 60–70 grams of protein.

Examples of healthy protein options:
3 oz. lean chicken (27 grams of protein)
3 oz. tuna (23 grams of protein)
3 oz. lean beef (25 grams of protein)
1 cup low-fat cottage cheese (28 grams of protein)
8 oz. low-fat milk (8 grams of protein)
8 oz. low-fat yogurt (9 grams of protein)
½ cup raw tofu (10 grams of protein)
1 whole egg (6 grams of protein)
1 cup boiled lentils (18 grams of protein)
1 cup cooked garbanzo beans (12 grams of protein)
¼ cup wheat germ (7 grams of protein)

Fat

It's important to watch what kinds of fat you're consuming through pregnancy, while breastfeeding, and when you're trying to slim down after your baby arrives.

First, let's talk about which fats you should avoid. Less than 10 percent of the total calories in your diet should come from saturated fats, which can

HEALTHY SNACKS

Three snacks a day in between meals will keep your sugar levels from falling and help you consume all the nutrients needed for you and your baby. A few tips for easy snacking:

- Buy small plastic bags so that you can portion out the correct amount of snacks (nuts, fruit, whole-grain crackers, and pretzels) and take them with you when you're on the go.
- Look for small plastic dishes that have a spot in their lids for dips. They're a great way to make snacks like carrots and hummus or peanut butter and whole wheat crackers portable.
- Try preparing all your snacks on the weekend so that you can just pick them up and go without any fuss.
- See Chapter 10 for yummy snack selections.

increase cholesterol levels and up your risk of heart disease, so make an effort to limit your consumption of whole milk, butter, cheese, and fatty meats. You should also steer clear of trans fats, which are those that have been altered by food manufacturers in order to give commercial snack foods a longer shelf life. They're found in fried foods such as French fries as well as in vegetable shortening and some margarines. Food with the words "hydrogenated vegetable oils," "partially hydrogenated oils," and "shortening" on their labels are a sign of these bad fats.

It's important to avoid trans fats as much as possible since research suggests that they may impair your body's ability to produce essential fatty acids, which your baby needs both while in utero and when nursing. Other studies suggest that while you're pregnant some fatty acids may pass through the placenta and harm your baby, and that post-pregnancy they can get into your breast milk.

The American Academy of Pediatrics suggests avoiding nuts while pregnant and breastfeeding if nut allergies run in your family.

My favorite brand of organic flaxseeds and fish oil supplements is Barlean's (www.barleans.com). This company's products are available at most health-food stores. Recently Barlean's released a new product, Omega Swirl, which is flaxseed oil emulsified in a strawberry and banana flavor. I give my kids a teaspoon every day, and it's so yummy that they think it's dessert and actually ask for more!

Though it's important to get your nutrients primarily from food, your prenatal vitamin can be a great way to get many of the recommended doses of nutrients that your growing baby needs. (Take it with meals to avoid nausea.)

That said, it's important to get your fill of healthy fats. Opt for mono-unsaturated fats found in foods like olive oil and polyunsaturated fats found in foods like sunflower oil. Some fatty acids, such as omega-3, omega-6, and docosahexaenoic acid (DHA), are crucial during pregnancy and while breastfeeding in order for your baby's brain, cells, and retinal, nervous, and cardiovascular systems to develop properly. Recent studies have found that children whose mothers ate fish containing these fatty acids at least three times a week while pregnant had better social, behavior, communication, and fine-motor skills than children whose mothers did not. And other research suggests that DHA helps with post-partum depression if consumed during pregnancy and afterward. Get these healthy fats in foods like salmon, herring, sardines, avocados, walnuts, wheat germ, canola oil, flaxseeds, or eggs enriched with omega-3s or

DHA. Nuts like almonds, cashews, peanuts, and walnuts, as well as sunflower, pumpkin, and sesame seeds, are also a great source. I love to get my daily fill by sprinkling a teaspoon of freshly ground flaxseeds (keep them refrigerated) on my cereal or mixing them in my smoothies.

Post-pregnancy you may be tempted to cut fats out of your diet completely because you think they'll, well, make you fat. But that's one of the biggest nutrition myths out there. As long as you choose healthy fats, enjoy them.

Calcium

Your baby needs calcium to build bones and strong muscles, and especially for his or her heart. If you don't consume enough, your baby's bones steal calcium from *your* bones, which ups your risk of osteoporosis later in life. Interestingly, your body absorbs calcium better when you're pregnant and nursing, so the recommended daily amount is the same as when you're not pregnant (1,000 to 1,200 milligrams). There are many great sources of calcium, like cheese, milk, and yogurt. (I love YoMommy organic yogurts, which are fortified with folic acid, added DHA, and vitamin D.) And yes, the occasional ice cream counts, too. Here are a few things to note about calcium:

- Many prenatal vitamins contain calcium; those that contain calcium citrate are absorbed best.
- Getting adequate amounts of vitamin D is important in order for the body to absorb calcium. Your prenatal vitamin should have this, too, but double check.
- If you're taking calcium and iron tablets, take them at different times of the day so they'll be better absorbed by the body.

Examples of good calcium options:
1 cup low-fat milk (300 milligrams) (Your required daily amount is
    equal to 3–4 glasses of milk.)
1 cup firm tofu (200 milligrams)
1 cup yogurt (300–400 milligrams)
1 cup broccoli (100 milligrams)
2 oz. cheese (400 milligrams)

Iron

When you're pregnant, your blood volume increases by 50 percent! As a result of all this extra blood circulating in your body, you will need to get more iron into your diet so that you don't become anemic. (Symptoms of anemia include paleness, dizziness, fatigue, shortness of breath, and heart palpitations.) Though it's critical to get enough iron throughout your pregnancy, it's especially critical in the third trimester, when your baby's body is storing iron to use during his or her first six months of life.

If you're breastfeeding, your iron requirement will actually decrease postpartum because breastfeeding often puts a halt to your period, allowing your body to store iron. However, if you do start to menstruate or aren't breastfeeding, your need for iron will return to regular pre-pregnancy levels. Try foods like chicken, beef, pork, eggs, tofu, dried apricots, raisins, dates, prunes, spinach, kidney beans, chickpeas, and soybeans. Just note that if you choose plant sources of iron, eating it with vitamin C can help your body absorb it better. So wash those raisins down with a glass of orange juice or add grapefruit wedges to your spinach salad.

> Red meat contains iron, which you need postpartum because you may lose a lot of blood during delivery. Grass-fed red meat is the best choice, but it's expensive and not always available, so choose the leanest meats that you can find to keep your intake of saturated fats low. Then trim any visible fat when you get home.

Examples of other good iron-rich foods:
1 cup General Mills Total Breakfast Cereal (about 23 milligrams)
1 cup soybeans (about 9 milligrams)
1 cup spinach (about 6.5 milligrams)

Folic Acid

Folic acid is vital for the healthy development of your baby's spinal cord and red blood cells, while a diet that's deficient in folate may cause spina bifida, a serious neural tube defect that can occur in the first trimester when the spinal cord develops. Though it's crucial to make sure your prenatal vitamin has at least 0.4 milligrams, which equals 400 micrograms of folate, the American Dietetic Association recommends that at least 200 additional micrograms should come from foods. Terrific sources include dark, leafy

> Unless prescribed by your doctor, never consume an excess amount of one particular vitamin, as it can be harmful to your baby. When in doubt, always consult with your MD.

vegetables like spinach, collard greens, and Romaine lettuce as well as broccoli, asparagus, and fortified breads, pastas, rice, and cereals.

Examples of folate-rich options:
1 cup cooked lentils (358 micrograms)
1 cup cooked chickpeas (160 micrograms)
1 cup cooked spinach (263 micrograms)
1 cup orange juice (109 micrograms)
1 cup peas (101 micrograms)
½ cup broccoli (39 micrograms)
1 cup strawberries (26 micrograms)

Choline

We haven't heard much about choline until recently, when several animal studies found that it may help promote brain development and memory function. A recommended daily allowance (RDA) for this nutrient has yet to be established, but the National Academy of Sciences recommends that pregnant women get 450 milligrams daily for "adequate intake." You can find it in eggs, beef, and chicken livers.

DID YOU KNOW?

Feeling stressed during pregnancy can impact your diet. A study at Johns Hopkins University found that women who were overtired, fatigued, and stressed out ate more unhealthy foods like candy and cookies and fewer nutrient-rich foods like fruits, veggies, and beans than women who were well rested and not stressed. If stress sends you to the fridge, try other calming activities, such as taking a walk or a bath, calling a close friend, or treating yourself to a manicure or pedicure.

Phytochemicals

Phytochemicals are plant chemicals that have an array of benefits and disease-fighting properties. Most of them act as antioxidants, which means that they protect our cells against damage and diseases. Others, like isoflavones, which are found in soy foods, mimic estrogen and are helpful in warding off menopausal symptoms and osteoporosis. Some experts also believe that consuming phytochemicals can be a natural way to regulate your hormones—something that's priceless during the nine months when your hormones go haywire, or postpartum when the baby blues or depression can take hold of you. There are many phytochemicals, and the best way to get them is by loading up on fruits like blueberries, cranberries, cherries, and apples; veggies like cauliflower, cabbage, carrots, and broccoli; and soy foods, whole grains, beans, herbs, and herbal teas.

Water

Staying hydrated is important while you're pregnant and post-pregnancy to help ward off morning sickness, constipation, and fatigue. Water is also necessary for the amniotic fluid that your baby floats in for nine months, while a lack of water can cause early contractions. You need eight 8-ounce glasses of water a day. An easy way to know that you're drinking enough is if your urine is light in color not bright yellow.

Tap water is generally safe, but if you suspect that your plumbing may be old with lead pipes, have the lead levels in your water supply checked first. (Women with long-term lead exposure are at risk of miscarriage and still births, and their babies may have long-term learning disabilities, among other negative impacts.) Invest in a purifying system, and before drinking tap water, let it run for a while. This way the water that's been sitting in the pipes for a few hours will flush away.

Essential Vitamins

Vitamin A

Betacarotene, found in fruits and veggies and converted into vitamin A, plays a vital role in the growth of healthy tissues and cells and is an antioxidant that protects you and your baby against cell damage. Great sources of this nutrient include leafy green veggies, citrus fruits, sweet potatoes, carrots, spinach, and milk, which is usually fortified with vitamin A. One word of caution: Large doses of vitamin A (10,000 IU or more) from supplements have been found to cause birth defects. However, you usually don't have to worry about getting too much from food or from your prenatal vitamins (most contain around 500 IU, which is well below the upper limit).

Vitamin D

This nutrient helps the body absorb calcium and distribute it to the bones. Research shows that vitamin D deficiency during pregnancy may cause soft bones to form in your baby's skull as well as dental problems. Though about 15 minutes of daily sun exposure can help your body produce the amount of vitamin D needed, the potential skin-cancer and sun-damage risk from UV rays may make some women wary of this option. However, I personally think the benefits are far greater than any negative issues, especially if you combine it with a nice walk around the block. Unfortunately, there are only a few foods—such as salmon and other oily fish—that contain vitamin D, so look for those that are fortified with it, such as milk and cereal bars.

If you like juice, make sure it's 100 percent fruit juice, and limit yourself to only 8 ounces a day, because the calories in juice can add up. Though a cup of orange juice contains about 207 percent of your RDA for vitamin C, it also has 111 calories. A cranberry juice of the same size contains 149 percent of your RDA for vitamin C and 144 calories.

Vitamin C

This powerful antioxidant helps strengthen the immune system, fight fatigue, and keep bones and joints strong. It's also vital for vegetarians because it helps the body absorb iron from plant sources. Our bodies are unable to store vitamin C, so it's critical that you eat vitamin C–rich foods daily. Though vitamin supplements are a good source, experts believe that fresh is best, so try to eat strawberries, citrus fruits (which may also help with morning sickness), broccoli, spinach, tomatoes, and red peppers. In fact, just one orange or two-thirds of a cup of strawberries meets your daily requirement.

B Vitamins

These important vitamins help with the release of energy from foods, something that's important for the growth of your baby. They also help to maintain the nervous system, to form healthy red blood cells, and to promote healthy skin and eyes. These vitamins are found in all food groups—whole grains, lentils, seafood, poultry, and nuts are all good sources—except veggies. This is why vegetarians or vegans who may not get an adequate amount of vitamin B12 in their diet are encouraged to take a supplement. (See also section "Folic Acid" earlier in this chapter. Folic acid is one of the B vitamins and is especially important during pregnancy.)

Zinc

Your body needs zinc for the production, repair, and functioning of DNA and to support your immune system, but it's also involved in all the phases of your baby's growth. In fact, studies have found that women with low levels have smaller babies and may deliver preterm. While you're pregnant, you will need 12 milligrams of zinc daily. If you're breastfeeding, this increases to 14 milligrams for the first six months, because your baby is actually draining your body's supply (which is why it's advised to pay careful attention to meeting this requirement). It's likely that your prenatal vitamin will contain your daily amount, and if you continue to take it post-pregnancy then you're covered. Good food choices are fortified cereals, red meat, poultry, seafood, nuts, dairy products, seeds, wheat germ, and whole grains. The National Academy of Sciences recommends zinc supplements of no more than 15 milligrams daily without medical supervision.

TABLE 5.1: ESSENTIAL NUTRIENTS THROUGH PREGNANCY AND BEYOND

NUTRIENTS	RDA FOR PREGNANCY	RDA FOR LACTATION	FOOD SOURCES
Protein	60–70 grams	70 grams	Meat, dairy, beans, eggs
Calcium	1,200 milligrams	1,200 milligrams	Milk, yogurt, cheese, dark leafy veggies
Iron	30 milligrams	15 milligrams	Lean red meat, spinach, whole grains, enriched breads and cereals
Folic acid	400 micrograms	400 micrograms	Green leafy veggies, nuts, legumes, enriched cereals and breads, yellow and orange fruits and veggies
Vitamin A	770 micrograms	1,300 micrograms	Green leafy veggies, milk, carrots, sweet potatoes
Vitamin D	5 micrograms	5 micrograms	Fortified milk, sun exposure
Vitamin C	85 milligrams	120 milligrams	Citrus fruits, broccoli, tomatoes
Thiamine (B1)	1.4 milligrams	1.6 milligrams	Whole-grain enriched breads and cereals, milk, fish, lean meats
Riboflavin (B2)	1.4 milligrams	1.6 milligrams	Whole-grain enriched breads and cereals, green leafy veggies, liver
Niacin (B3)	18 milligrams	20 milligrams	Whole-grain enriched breads and cereals, poultry, fish, liver, meat
Pyridoxine (B6)	1.9 milligrams	1.9 milligrams	Whole grains, enriched cereals and breads, beef, liver, pork, ham, bananas, soy-based meat substitutes
B12	2.6 micrograms	2.8 micrograms	Liver, milk, poultry
Iodine	220 micrograms	290 micrograms	Milk and other dairy products, spinach, kale, turnips, salmon and sardines with bones, iodized salt
Phosphorus	700 milligrams	700 milligrams	Dairy, meat, fish, legumes, whole grains or enriched breads and cereals
Magnesium	2.0 milligrams	2.6 milligrams	Whole grains, enriched cereals and breads, legumes, milk, green veggies, nuts, meat
Zinc	11 milligrams	12 milligrams	Whole grains, enriched cereals and breads, fish, meat, liver

TROUBLESHOOTING COMMON DIGESTIVE PROBLEMS

Curing Constipation

Constipation and pregnancy go hand-in-hand thanks to the hormonal changes that relax the digestive tract and slow your system down. The uterus may also place pressure on the bowels, making it harder to pass a stool.

- Water will help keep stool soft, making it easier to pass.
- Eating plenty of fiber helps your stool pass through the gastrointestinal track. Aim for 20–35 grams a day from foods like whole grains, fruits, veggies, and legumes (such as lentils).
- Exercise and light physical activity helps to keep you regular by moving the bowels.

Avoiding Heartburn

Heartburn is most common in the third trimester for two reasons. First, the uterus presses against the stomach, forcing its contents and gastric acids to move up the esophagus. Second, pregnancy hormones relax the valve that separates the stomach and the esophagus, making it easy for gastric acid to move upward and cause discomfort. To avoid heartburn, try the following techniques:

- Eat small meals (as opposed to large ones) and eat slowly to reduce the amount of food in your stomach at one time.
- Sit upright and don't lie down right after eating so that less food moves up into the esophagus.
- Avoid spicy, fatty, greasy foods as well as chocolate and caffeine as they have been proven to aggravate heartburn.

DID YOU KNOW?

Having a healthy diet while pregnant may increase the chances that your child will eat more than mac-n-cheese and chicken nuggets later in life. Research shows that the flavors found in a pregnant woman's amniotic fluid and breast milk may affect her child's food preferences. In one study, moms who ate lots of carrot juice and fruits during pregnancy were more likely to have kids who liked these foods than those who didn't eat them.

Cravings and Aversions

Pickles and ice cream may be an old cliché (and I've yet to meet any woman who's actually eaten them). But a deep desire for certain foods (often in strange combinations) is commonplace during pregnancy. In fact, you'll be surprised by some of the things that you long for. I constantly craved mashed potatoes and bagels with cream cheese, which are foods that I hadn't eaten in years. One theory about pregnancy cravings is that they may be your body's way of telling you that you're deficient in a particular nutrient. Yet, since not all cravings are particularly healthy, it's unclear whether this is true.

On the flip side of cravings is food aversions, and you may find yourself turned off during pregnancy by foods you used to love. I had a friend who was so averse to pizza that seeing the word on a restaurant sign made her feel sick! Some women have been known to crave non-food items such as dirt, clay, plaster, laundry starch, and many other substances. This condition is referred to as pica, and some experts say it's a symptom of an iron deficiency. Try not to give in to your cravings (at least most of the time) unless they're for food that's going to deliver all those much-needed nutrients and minerals. You can keep cravings at bay by having healthy snacks at hand all the time.

TABLE 5.2: FOOD PORTION RECOMMENDATIONS

FOOD GROUP	DAILY AMOUNT	PORTION SIZE
Protein	6–8 servings a day	1 oz. fish or chicken
Dairy	4–5 servings a day	1 cup low-fat skim milk or 1 oz. cheese
Grains	6–11 servings a day	1 slice whole-wheat bread or ½ cup brown rice
Fruits and vegetables	5–9 servings a day	1 medium apple or ½ cup spinach

Note: See Chapter 10 for a list of foods in each category and portion exchanges.

Team Mallett Success Story

Veronica Dowdy, 40, Los Angeles, CA

Lost

13 pounds

5 dress sizes

30 total inches

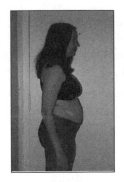
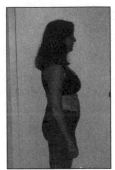

Before   After

• • • • •

Veronica's baby was already six months old and Veronica was still wearing her maternity clothes. "I had all these beautiful clothes in my closet and stored in boxes that I couldn't fit into," she says. "I felt out of shape, unattractive, and had no energy." This was quite a change from the woman Veronica was before she became a mom. Most of her life she'd been a size four and very active. "In fact, I was training for a marathon and had just run 20 miles when I found out that I was expecting," she says. When she heard that Tracey was looking for women to join the Super Fit Mama plan, Veronica jumped at the chance. "I really needed the challenge and was excited about the opportunity to work with an expert," she recalls.

At times Veronica's motivation to work out wavered, but she enlisted her husband to help. "He playfully held my favorite pair of jeans in front of me to remind me why I was working out," she says. Even when life happens—like her daughter gets sick, and exercising and eating right are the last things she has the time or energy for—Veronica reminds herself that "when I work out, I am at my best. I have more energy and feel healthy and that allows me to be available to my family," she says.

The diet part of the Super Fit Mama program was surprisingly easy for Veronica to incorporate into her life. "It's simple and not too restricted," she says. "I always hated counting calories, but this plan makes it a cinch to keep track of what I'm eating. I'm also amazed at how satisfied I feel with the food plan and how something like plain Greek yogurt blended with frozen mangos can satisfy my craving for dessert." Veronica also kept her diet on track by preparing her meals in advance. "During the evening, I'd make meals for the next day," she says. "That helped me not go overboard."

Even after just a few weeks on the program, Veronica saw a change. "My face was thinner, my stomach started to disappear, and my arms looked shapelier again," she says. Now, months later, she feels better than ever and has a fabulous attitude. "I feel a lot more confident, sexier, and feminine, with energy and focus," she says. "I have had my lows and highs, but I don't kick myself when I'm down since I know that we all go through that. I think we all want to be perfect wives, moms, and partners and perfect with our workouts and diets. But what I've realized is that being "perfect" is impossible, so I kept it simple and simply celebrated each pound I lost."

CHAPTER 6

THE FIRST
SIX WEEKS
POSTPARTUM

So you've brought your beautiful baby home and spent the first days in awe of this tiny new life that you brought into the world. If you're like me, you'll never quite get over that feeling. I remember those days like they were yesterday (hang on a second while I wipe a few tears away). One look at my daughter, and all the discomforts of pregnancy seemed worth it. I was amazed by everything about her, from her ruby-colored lips to her tiny fingers to her soft, protruding belly and chubby thighs. I couldn't believe she was mine. However, I was also amazed by my own chubby little thighs and rounded belly. I couldn't believe they were mine too!

I felt like a huge deflated balloon. I remember looking down at my once-firm abs and seeing only a sea of flab. What made matters worse was reading tabloids filled with stories about how some celebrity had a baby and was prancing around in her size 2 jeans in a matter of weeks. (First off, don't believe the hype—thanks to retouching, many of those celebrity photos have been magically revised. Secondly, most of us could slim down fast, too, if we had an on-call cook, trainer, nannies, and masseuse.) Still, like most women I knew, I wanted to have my beautiful baby and then slip right into my old body. We wish!

If this sounds like you, don't despair. Because the good news is that you can bounce back—just take a look at the forty-five women on Team Mallett. First things first: Put your pre-pregnancy clothes down and step away from the mirror. You JUST had a baby. Yes, your body created a little human being and housed him or her for nine months, so give yourself a break. Second, remember that it took you nine months to gain all that weight, so it's not going to magically disappear in nine minutes or nine days.

During these first six weeks, some of your weight is going to naturally come off as your body recovers. Whoo hoo! In those first weeks, I lost about 15 pounds. The way that weight breaks down varies from one woman to the next, but in general it consists of the baby (about 6.5–9 pounds), the placenta (about 1.5 pounds), the amniotic fluid (about 2 pounds), breast enlargement (about 1–3 pounds; too bad you can't keep those!), uterus enlargement (about 2 pounds), fat stores (about 6–8 pounds), increased blood and fluid volume (about 5–7 pounds). Nursing will expedite this process and help your uterus shrink, but it's a big myth that breastfeeding alone is enough to get your pre-pregnancy body back. Unfortunately, there is no magic bullet to weight loss and you still have to eat a healthy diet and get some exercise (sorry!).

EXERCISING AFTER BABY

Here's more good news: That postnatal exercise will do more than help you slim down. It will also speed up your recovery process and provide the strength that your body needs to keep up with the hectic schedule of caring for your newborn. Having a formal plan like the Super Fit Mama Body After Baby program, presented in the coming chapters, is a great way to get started. Proof comes from a study at Saint Louis University, which found that women who were on a structured exercise program postpartum lost more weight than those who weren't on such a plan. Another study found that combining exercise with a healthy diet (also presented in the upcoming chapters) is a more effective way to slim down after pregnancy than dieting without breaking a sweat.

Of course, you should always consult with your doctor or midwife before starting any exercise program, and they may ask you to wait until your six-week postpartum checkup so they can see how you're doing. The kind of delivery you had will also determine how quickly you can resume exercise. If you had a vaginal delivery, it's likely that your doctor will give you the okay sooner than if you had a C-section (in which case you'll typically have to wait about six to eight weeks). However, it's actually recommended that you strengthen the transverse abdominals and

C-SECTIONS 101

A C-section is abdominal surgery—something that most people forget—and the incision through the abdominal wall means you have to modify some of your regular activities to help ease the pain. Here are some tips to help get you through the first few days:

1. Coughing can cause pain where the incision is as it stresses the abdominals and the pelvic floor. Place a rolled-up towel or soft pillow over the incision and slightly lean forward, and then cough.
2. When feeding the baby, place a soft pillow over your abdomen or use a large Boppy cushion (the feeding and support version). These can be found in most stores that sell supplies for babies and new moms, or see www.boppy.com. This is perfect for C-sections as it protects the incision.
3. When riding in a car, place a folded towel or a pillow on your abdomen to protect yourself from the seat belt.
4. Never jack-knife (sit straight up) out of bed. Always roll over to the side and push yourself up with your hands, preventing strain on weak abdominal and pelvic floor muscles, and of course the incision.

pelvic floor within the first two days after a normal vaginal delivery so that you can restore the muscle tone that helps these areas perform their supportive functions (as long as there is no pain associated with doing so). If you've had a C-section, you can try walking within the first week, something that can help decrease the chance of thrombophlebitis (formation of blood clots) and improve bowel and bladder function. It will also help alleviate those gas pains that are common after surgery.

Regardless of which type of delivery you've had, the key is to be patient with yourself. Your body requires rest and recovery. If you rush into strenuous exercise and aren't fully healed, you'll set yourself back even further. I was so obsessed about losing the weight after my son was born that I decided to go out for a 45-minute run six weeks postpartum. I ended up falling over because my legs were too tired, spraining my ankle, and straining my hip flexors. Another reason that you need to be careful about exercising postpartum is that your joints and ligaments will still be loose for about three to five months, thanks to the pregnancy hormone relaxin. (This time frame is even longer if you continue to breastfeed past that time.) Also, right now the hormone levels in your body are trying to get back to normal, which will leave you feeling really tired. Tack on the stress and effort of dealing with a newborn, and it's easy to see why you're exhausted.

If you exercised throughout your pregnancy, had a normal vaginal delivery, and have consent from your MD, you can safely perform the exercises in this chapter plus light exercise such as walking and stretching within a few days after delivery. It's still not advised to do any kind of high-impact aerobic activity, which can cause hemorrhaging (a little bleeding is expected after delivery, but too much activity can make this problematic). Remember, patience is the key! Getting back into shape should begin slowly. Even if you only walk around your backyard or the block, it's a start. Take time to get in tune with your body.

Lastly, remember to enjoy this time with your baby. It may be a cliché, but it's true: The time flies! You have created the miracle of life. A little extra weight is a small price to pay for that bundle of joy. Also, I promise that you *will* lose the baby fat and get your body back, but you won't get back these early newborn days.

Seventy-two percent of women in the United States breastfeed right after the birth of their babies, but this number drops to 40 percent by three months postpartum. By six months postpartum, just 14 percent of new moms are still breastfeeding.

FREQUENTLY ASKED POST-PREGNANCY QUESTIONS

If you're like most of the women on Team Mallett, you probably have tons of questions at this point. Here are the most common questions I've been asked by new moms, and, more importantly, the answers!

1. Why are my abs separated? I look like I have a melon tummy!
By far, my abs were the most bothersome part of my post-baby body. I wished that someone had warned me that my abs would look like Play-Doh after delivery. Not only was there that little pooch from my uterus and stretched muscles, but there was mush that hung over my waistband and seemed to jiggle when I walked. I wasn't asking for a six-pack (or even a four-pack), but I was longing for a flatter middle. You may feel the same way, but caution and patience are required before jumping back into an exercise program, especially with your stretched-out abdominals and pelvic floor.

As described earlier, during pregnancy you'll probably notice a dark line going down the center of your abs. It's called the linea nigra. Take a look at this dark line and you'll likely notice that there is a recti muscle to the right and the left. These muscles attach to thin fibrous horizontal bands with about a one-half-inch gap. This seam is very vulnerable to separation during pregnancy thanks to the pressure of the growing baby in the uterus, which leans against the front wall of the abdominals. This pressure, combined with hormonal changes, excessive weight gain, and bearing down through labor, can force this gap to open near the belly button like a zipper. This separation can range in size from 2 to 20 centimeters in width and 12 to 15 centimeters in length. The separation itself is called *diastasis recti,* and studies show that 37 percent of women who have one pregnancy experience this condition while 67 percent of women who have had multiple pregnancies do so.

Other factors that predispose you to diastasis recti are obesity, having a large baby, excessive uterine fluid, and weak abdominals prior to pregnancy. The most common symptoms are low back, buttock, and/or hip pain and a vertical bulge in the middle of your abdomen when standing or sitting (which turns into a bulge when you're lying on the floor and lift your head like you would in an abdominal crunch). Because sheer force can make this separation—and its accompanying bulge—even worse, it's important to monitor it before you do any abdominal exercises, especially rotation activities, or even getting up from a horizontal position (roll to the side before rising). Also, avoid exercises where you're lying on your back and lowering your legs (such as straight leg raises, dipping the toes, single leg stretches, the 100s).

It's crucial to close the gap, because when the rectus abdominals are separated it leaves your pelvis very unstable, which can eventually lead to lower-back and hip pain and will make it hard to strengthen and flatten your abs. In the worst-case scenario, this separation can result in a hernia. See Chapter 2 for diagrams of normal abdominal muscles and separated ones.

What to Do

Before doing any strenuous abdominal work, it's important to gauge the amount of separation you have. To do so, use the following test.

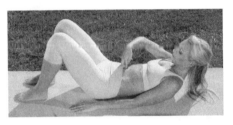

- Lay on your back with your knees bent and your fingers placed above your belly button.
- Lift your head, neck, and shoulders off the floor and press your fingers firmly down. Feel to see if you have a gap in between your abs.
- If you do feel a gap, use your fingers to measure the size of the separation.
- Repeat the test, but this time place your fingers below the belly button.
- If either gap is the width of two or three fingers or more, do the towel abs exercise below and only perform core-strengthening exercises in this book that are marked with an asterisk. With these exercises you can work on correcting the separation before you move on to more strenuous abdominal work. The exercises marked with an asterisk will train the abdominals back together again, creating a stronger, stable spine.

Abdominal Wraps

Many women, especially celebrities, swear that wearing an abdominal wrap around the midsection after birth really helps their abdominals get back to pre-pregnancy state quicker. I agree that wrapping your abs will force your muscles to come back together if they're separated and can help to stop the condition from getting worse. It will also give you that extra back support and a natural reminder to activate your abs throughout the day. I personally like the Belly Bandit (www.bellybandit.com).

Note: Do not perform any of the abdominal exercises below while wearing the wrap. The wrap is a tool that can help you recover faster, but it is not a substitute for exercising caution when working out the midsection.

Towel abs exercise

Muscles targeted: Abdominals

Reps: 2 sets of 10 reps (work up to 40 reps per day as you get stronger)

A. Lay on your back with your knees bent and your heels in line with the sit bones (those bony parts you feel under your pelvis you when you sit down). Wrap a towel around your midsection and cross the towel over your abs (holding it at each end).

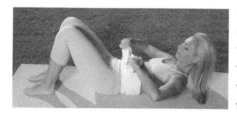

B. Lift your head, neck, and shoulders off the floor, exhale, and draw your abdominals in toward the spine while tilting your pelvis up. This will activate the transverse abdominals. Then, pull the towel tight. This will pull the abs together, retraining them to go back to their correct, functional position.

Modification: If your neck begins to ache, perform the exercise by lifting just your head and neck off the floor.

2. How come I leak every time I sneeze, cough, or laugh too hard?

This lovely post-pregnancy side effect, called *urinary incontinence* and experienced by 26 percent of women ages 30–39 after pregnancy, is the result of a weakened pelvic floor. (Other signs of pelvic floor dysfunction, as it's called, are urinary urgency and frequency, fecal incontinence, and pelvic organ prolapse and pain.) Before pregnancy, the pelvic floor muscles, which attach

Tracey's Tips

Keep monitoring the separation. Also, you don't need to do all your reps at the same time, but can spread them throughout the day. Until the abs are no more than two fingers' width apart, stay away from any strenuous abdominal work—especially rotational ab work, lifting heavy objects (only lift the weight of the baby), and leg lowering exercises—as this will make the separation worse.

Think about bringing your belly button toward your spine with everything you do, such as when you sneeze, cough, laugh, pick up your baby, get up and down, and exercise. If you can't hold your belly button to the spine when doing any activity, it's an indication that you shouldn't be doing that activity because you're probably forcefully pushing forward, making that separation larger.

at the pubic bone, tailbone, and sit bones, is relatively flat. After pregnancy and childbirth, it looks more like a sagging hammock. A weak pelvic floor is often associated with vaginal deliveries because of tearing during childbirth, episiotomies, and the use of forceps. However, it can also happen to women who have had C-sections—especially those who have spent many hours in labor. Studies suggest that even an elective C-section doesn't stop you from experiencing urinary incontinence.

Exercise is key to helping your pelvic floor recover. In fact, it's probably the most important muscle to strengthen after pregnancy because this area has lots of key responsibilities: It supports the vital organs in the pelvic area, is used for delivery and sex (orgasms), impacts urinary and bowel control, and provides core support for activities such as laughing, coughing, and sneezing as well as abdominal workouts, high-impact aerobics, and lifting your baby!!

What to Do

Treatment includes bladder retraining, strengthening of the pelvic floor muscles utilizing biofeedback, and hip and core strengthening. Right now, here's what you can do on your own. To help strengthen this area, try doing 20 reps of pelvic floor exercises (a.k.a. Kegel exercises) three times per day. Also, do them when performing activities such as lifting your baby, going from a seated to a standing position, or going up and down stairs. These can be done anywhere and are essential for achieving a strong, stable pelvic area.

3. Why is my back constantly aching?

Despite all the joys, motherhood can be a real pain in the back. An amazing 62 percent of women experience back pain postpartum, and only 37 percent of this resolves itself within eighteen months. Lower back issues are primarily caused by tight muscles in the lumbar spine and pelvis, weak and stretched-out abdominals, and diastasis recti. Tight hip flexors and hamstrings can also pull on the pelvis causing additional pain and discomfort. And lastly, the pelvis, which has stretched out to make room for baby, is still very unstable and slowly moving back together, and this can increase any pain. Add carrying, cuddling, and feeding your baby, and you've got a recipe for aches and pains in your upper back, neck, and shoulders.

What to Do

The core exercises in this chapter will help you regain strength and support in the core, and the stretches will help release tension in the lower back and pelvic region. Learning correct body mechanics for your daily activities (see sidebar on page 125, "Daily Activity Dos and Don'ts") will help reduce unnecessary back strain. Of course, if your pain persists, you may need to be assessed by a physical therapist.

4. Why do I look like the Hunchback of Notre Dame and continually have shoulder and neck pain?

Take a glance at the other moms around you and you'll see that you're certainly not alone in your hunched back state. Of course, this isn't surprising, considering all the extra weight your body has carried while pregnant and the natural mechanical strain of that growing belly. Also, throughout pregnancy our bodies will compensate in order to be able to balance and function, but not necessarily in a good way. Our muscles get fatigued and underused, especially the upper back muscles, which is

---

TIPS FROM THE PROS: A GUIDE TO PELVIC FLOOR DYSFUNCTION AFTER DELIVERY

Laura Horn, MPT, Women's Health Physical Therapist

How do you know if you're experiencing bladder or pelvic floor dysfunction? Ask yourself the following questions; if you answer yes to one or more and these symptoms do not resolve within six months postpartum, talk with your OB-GYN. You may want to ask for a referral to a women's health physical therapist.

- Do you urinate more than six to eight times every twenty-four hours? Do you do so more frequently than every two hours? If so, you may have *problems with frequency*.
- Do you feel a strong, uncontrollable urge to urinate even if your bladder is not full? If so, you may be experiencing problems with *urgency*.
- Do you awake from sleep with the strong urge to urinate more than two or three times a night? If so, you may have *nocturia*.
- Do you leak urine when you cough, sneeze, laugh, lift your baby, chase your kids, or exercise? If so, you may have *stress urinary incontinence*.
- Do you experience a strong urge to urinate followed by an involuntary leakage of urine on the way to the bathroom? Is your leakage triggered by cold temperatures, running water, or placing your key in the door? If so, you may be experiencing *urge incontinence*.
- Do you feel a sensation of pelvic heaviness or pressure often with prolonged standing or during exertion (i.e., lifting or holding baby, or straining with a bowel movement)? If so, this may be *pelvic organ prolapse*.

Contact the American Physical Therapy Association Women's Health Section to find a women's health specialist close to you (www.womenshealthapta.org).

why we paid a lot of attention to keeping the back strong in the pre-pregnancy workout.

Once you have your little bundle of joy, you may shed your pregnancy pounds, but you're now toting your baby around in your arms, plus you have the added weight of all that breast milk, which inevitably causes postural changes that weaken the upper back muscles and can cause back strain. Even I (otherwise known as "Miss Flat Chest") went up three cup sizes and remained there until I weaned my baby a year later. You're also bent over when nursing your baby, getting in and out of the car, and carrying your diaper bag. All this can cause the spine to curve forward in a hunched position and give you shoulder and neck spasms. You're going to need a strong upper back to counteract these effects.

BABY CARRIERS

Baby carriers are a great way to balance the weight of the baby and help prevent injuries. Newborns love being held close to the heart and the calming movement that simulates their life in vitro, plus you'll love that little warm body snuggled up against you (and you can actually get some tasks done!). There are so many on the market these days, but I love the Ergobaby (www.ergobaby.com). Not only is the back-saving design pure genius, but I love that it can be adjusted as the baby gets bigger and can be worn front, side, and back.

What to Do

Try using a pillow on your lap while breastfeeding and make sure you're wearing a nursing bra that fits you well. Also, check to make sure that your baby sling or carrier is properly adjusted so that you're not hunched over or in pain while using it. The towel stretches and spine stretch in this chapter will help your posture. They release tight chest muscles, enabling your shoulders to move back into their proper alignment, and counteract all of the bent-over postures you may find yourself in throughout the day. You can also decrease the pain by be-

BACK AND BODY SAVING TIPS FOR NEW MOMS

By now, you've probably realized that having a baby doesn't just mean toting around the weight of the baby, but toting around all his or her paraphernalia, like the car seat, the stroller, and the diaper bag, as well. On top of all that, you're constantly picking your baby up off the floor and out of the crib, high-chair, and car. That's why it's so important to watch your body mechanics when lifting and carrying your little one and all his or her accessories.

Your pelvis is already loosey-goosey thanks to those hormones. Try to avoid balancing your baby on your hip. Though moms everywhere do this, it's the biggest contributing factor to lower back and hip issues post-pregnancy. New moms are also very susceptible to knee problems. The bottom line: Be aware of how you adjust your body to the new tasks of motherhood so that you can ward off injuries. (See sidebar on "Baby Carriers" for another important back-saving tip.)

coming more aware of your posture throughout the day and focusing on better body mechanics.

5. Why is my energy level so low? I feel so down all the time?

Give yourself a little break. You have pretty much run one marathon called pregnancy and are now starting your second one called motherhood. And since you're doing all this without much sleep or recovery, it would actually be strange if you *didn't* feel tired! (Don't believe those other new moms who say they're not exhausted.) Also, if you had a C-section, remember that this is a major surgery, so no wonder you're twice as drained. My biggest tip: Say yes to help. I know it's not easy, especially for us multitasking, do-it-yourself type gals, but accept it while you can get it. Your body needs time to rest and heal.

If you're feeling a little down, you're not alone. Your hormone levels are fluctuating, and this can take you on an emotional roller coaster and

DAILY ACTIVITY DOS & DON'TS

Don't bend over from the waist to pick up heavy objects. This places tremendous strain on the lower back and your stretched-out weak abs.

Do squat down to the floor while engaging your abdominals and keeping the spine nice and tall. Not only will your spine be more supported, but you will work your pelvic floor at the same time!

Don't hold the baby on one hip all the time.

Do switch from side to side to keep the weight distribution even, and try not to jut the hip out, but keep the pelvis in alignment. Ultimately, I suggest avoiding holding the baby on the hip at all if possible. Instead, hold him or her in the front and use a baby carrier or sling to distribute the baby's weight while keeping your hands free.

Don't jack-knife up from a lying-down position. This will place strain on the abdominal wall and can increase stretching of the central seam—especially if you have diastasis recti.

Do bring your knees toward your chest and roll onto your side to rise from a lying-down position, using your hands to push your upper body up to a seated position while drawing in your abdominals. Place your hands on the bed or floor, bend one leg at a time, and use your quads (one of the strongest muscles of the body) to extend your knees to a standing position.

Don't reach over from the hips to pull the baby and car seat out of the car.

Do stand as close as you can to the car and place one foot on the ledge of the car, or step all the way into the car with one foot and place your knee on the seat. You'll need to squat low if you have a sedan. Once you're in the car, disconnect the car seat from its base and pull your baby or the car seat close to your body as you contract the abs for support.

Caution: If you have just had a C-section, always follow the lifting precautions provided by your MD. Usually, doctors suggest that you lift nothing greater than your baby's weight, so just because you *can* get the baby in and out of the car doesn't mean you should pick up the baby with the added weight of the car seat.

bring out your crabby side. Many women experience some slight depression, often called the "baby blues" if it happens within those initial two to three weeks postpartum. In fact, it's estimated that up to 80 percent of new moms cry easily or feel super stressed during this time. Some common symptoms are mood swings, crying spells, loss of appetite, sleeping problems, and feelings of irritability, anxiety, and loneliness. You can help yourself by getting plenty of rest, talking to other new moms (moms' groups, classes, or message boards on parenting sites are great for this),

TIPS FROM THE PROS: BREASTFEEDING: STARTING OUT RIGHT

Dale Alleyne-Ho, Hon., E.C.E., CCBE, LE

Start ASAP. Attempt breastfeeding as soon after your baby's birth as possible. This is an ideal time because he or she is in the "quiet alert" (cuddly and still) stage and has not yet entered that "newborn sleep" stage. Early breastfeeding also promotes uterine contractions, which help to prevent postpartum hemorrhaging.

Feed frequently. This will help you establish and maintain your milk supply within the first few days and weeks of breastfeeding.

Position for success. Positioning your baby correctly at the breast during each feeding is especially important during the first few weeks and helps prevent common problems associated with breastfeeding, such as sore nipples. The most common positions include the "cradle hold," the "cross cradle hold," the "football hold," and the "side-lying" positions. The latter two are especially good if you've had a C-section because your baby's not resting on the incision.

Know a good latch when you see one. Making sure your baby is latching onto the nipple correctly can help you prevent any potential breastfeeding problems early on. A good latch means that your baby takes the entire nipple and as much of the breast into his mouth as necessary for the nipple to be at the very back of his mouth, near his throat. To start, your baby's mouth has to open very wide, with his tongue down and forward in order for it to lie underneath the nipple.

Soothe sore nipples. If your nipples hurt or baby is not latching well, it may be in your best interest to seek the help of a local La Leche League group leader, a certified lactation consultant, a public health nurse, your midwife, or a breastfeeding clinic (most often located in a hospital). Sore nipples can also be treated by exposing them to the air as often as possible and rubbing in a little breast milk after each feeding. Commercially sold nipple creams containing 100 percent pure lanolin are another alternative.

End engorgement. When the breasts become very full and often painful to the touch, it is called *engorgement.* Most mothers experience this when their milk first comes in, but engorgement can also occur much later on, such as when your baby suddenly begins to sleep for a longer stretch of time without a feeding. Engorged breasts can make latching your baby onto the breast quite a task, and chances are that your baby will get very frustrated! Ice packs can be applied to the breasts between feedings to relieve any swelling, and a warm washcloth or shower can help with your milk flow. Try hand expressing a little milk before attempting to latch baby onto the breast.

Deal with plugged ducts. To the touch, a plugged duct may feel like a tender lump in the breast. Apply either a heating pad or a hot washcloth to the affected area and encourage your newborn to feed frequently on the affected side while you massage the lump in order to get the milk flowing again. However, if you are experiencing flu-like symptoms and have a fever, you may have a breast infection. In this case, you may see a red, sore area on the breast. Contact your health-care provider, who may prescribe antibiotic treatment.

and doing whatever makes you relax, be it a long walk, brunch with a friend, or watching your favorite funny movie.

However, if these feelings last longer than two to three weeks or come and go, or you feel a really deep sadness or have thoughts of despair, anxiety, serious mood swings, loss of interest in things you used to enjoy, or thoughts about hurting your baby or yourself, you may be experiencing a more serious form of the blues called "postpartum depression." At this time it's important to talk to your MD as soon as possible. And please, don't be embarrassed to bring it up. Doctors see this often and can really help you feel better. If you feel uncomfortable, take your husband or friend along and have them get the conversation rolling. You can also check out a resource like Postpartum Support International (PSI) (see www.ppmdsupport.com).

One way to tell the difference between baby blues and postpartum depression is that the latter keeps you from functioning well in your daily life. Support groups, counseling, and medication are treatments that have helped many, many women. Exercise can also help. A recent study from the University of Quebec in Montreal found that exercising at home reduced the feelings of mental and physical fatigue in women with postpartum depression.

BREASTFEEDING

The American Academy of Pediatrics suggests that babies be breastfed exclusively for the first six months and recommends that you keep breastfeeding for at least twelve months to reap the most benefit. But all those 2 A.M. feedings do more than nourish your baby (or give you gorgeous breasts); they can help you get your body back! Breastfeeding helps to stimulate the production of the hormone oxytocin, which causes the uterus to contract and shrink back to its pre-pregnancy size. In other words, nursing will help flatten your puffed-out belly and burn calories fast (an estimated 500 per day!).

Now, you may choose not to breastfeed and of course you can nourish your baby with some of the nutrient-rich formulas out there. However, studies do suggest that breastfeeding has benefits for your baby, including fewer stomach problems like diarrhea and respiratory illnesses, reduced risk of ear infections and anemia, enhanced immune system, improved cognitive skills, and improved sleep, just to name a few. There are also studies providing evidence that it can reduce mom's chances later on in life of having breast or ovarian cancer, diabetes, obesity, and osteoporosis, and it may reduce postpartum depression.

Though it's easier than making a bottle, breastfeeding is less precise, so women often wonder if their baby is getting enough milk. Your baby should be gaining weight, and by day three of breastfeeding, you should be changing about four wet diapers daily. Within a week, your baby should have about six to eight wet diapers daily.

Something else you may be worried about is how exercising affects breastfeeding. When you're exercising hard, such as running, your body creates a by-product called lactic acid that is thought to change the flavor of your breast milk. If I exercised before a feeding, my kids would fuss and not want to latch on. However, studies found that often it was the smell they didn't like, not the milk. I learned that cleaning my breasts with soap and water or showering before the feeding would remedy this problem.

POST-PREGNANCY EXERCISES

The following exercises can be done one to two days after delivery with the consent of your MD or a health-care provider. However, if you've had a C-section, talk to your doctor first, because you may need to wait a few weeks. Remember, always to listen to your body.

Time: About 5 minutes.

How to: Perform each exercise six times a week to build strength.

You'll need: A pillow.

1. Kegels

Kegels can be performed anywhere, but I recommend you take some time out of your busy day to do the following exercise to get the blood flow to the perineum to aid in the healing process.

Muscles targeted: Pelvic floor

Reps: 3 sets of 10 reps (spread throughout the day)

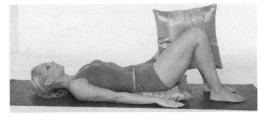

A. Begin by lying on your back with your knees bent, heels in line with your sit bones and a pillow underneath your hips to slightly elevate them.

B. Inhale through the nose, and on the exhale draw the pelvic floor up, hold for 5 seconds, then slowly release as you exhale. Progress to 10 seconds as you get stronger.

QUICK EXERCISE SAFETY TIPS

- Invest in a good support bra. Your breasts are going to be larger than normal from the milk production and will need a lot of extra support.
- Be careful about high-impact sports. As I mentioned, your body's ligaments and joints will still be lax thanks to hormones left over from pregnancy.
- Drink lots of water to replenish yourself, especially when breastfeeding.
- Listen to your body. If you're feeling tired, go easy on yourself. Try not to push yourself until you feel ready.
- If you start to feel lightheaded or nauseous, or notice a change in the color of your vaginal discharge, consult with your doctor. You may be exercising too strenuously.

2. Transverse breathing

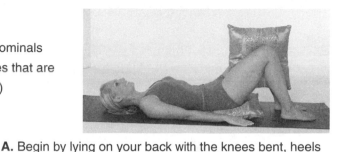

Muscles targeted: Transverse abdominals (deepest layer of abdominal muscles that are responsible for stabilizing the spine)

Reps: 10

A. Begin by lying on your back with the knees bent, heels in line with the sit bones, one pillow in between your knees and another under your hips.

B. Inhale through the nose, and as you exhale through the mouth draw your abs toward the spine without moving your pelvis. Perform 10 slow contractions and exhalations.

Tracey's Tips

As you inhale, feel the ribs expand. On the exhale the ribs will pull together and downward as you scoop the abdominals toward the spine, activating the transverse abdominals, while keeping the pelvis still. This exercise is harder than you may think after having a baby. You may not feel much happening, but if you persevere eventually the abs will start to respond.

Keep your glutes relaxed and let the abs do all the work. It's very easy to squeeze the glutes and let these stronger muscles do all the work. Focus on the abs titling the pelvis; there may not be much movement, as the abs are weak, but over time you will see a huge difference.

Walking while pushing your baby in the stroller is a great way to get out of the house and show off your beautiful newborn, and moving your body will boost circulation, which can speed the healing and recovery process. Start off gradually by going for short walks and taking rests when needed.

3. Pelvic tilts

Muscles targeted: Transverse abdominals and pelvic floor

Reps: 10

A. Begin by lying on your back with your knees bent, hip-width apart, and your heels in line with the sit bones. Your spine is in a neutral position and your arms are by your hips.

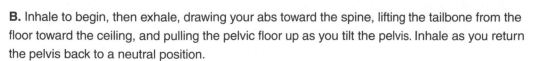

B. Inhale to begin, then exhale, drawing your abs toward the spine, lifting the tailbone from the floor toward the ceiling, and pulling the pelvic floor up as you tilt the pelvis. Inhale as you return the pelvis back to a neutral position.

4. Clams

Muscles targeted: Abdominals and glutes

Reps: 10 on each leg

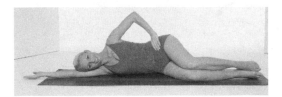

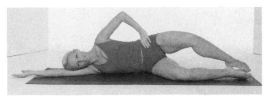

A. Begin by lying on your right hip with your knees bent, hips and knees stacked on top of each other. Your right arm is extended on the floor, with your right ear resting on the bicep, and your left hand is resting on the left hip.

B. Exhale and lift the top (left) knee toward the ceiling, keeping the heels together and the hips stacked, then inhale and lower the knee. Repeat to the other side.

Tracey's Tips

Keep your hips stacked and facing forward as you lift the knee. Imagine your femur (thigh bone) drawing in and up as your thigh lifts up. Lift your knee as high as you can without rotating the pelvis and lower spine.

5. Cat/Cow

Muscles targeted: Abdominals and lower back

Reps: 10

Tracey's Tips

Always try to engage the pelvic floor as you exhale, and keep the abdominals engaged even on the extension of the spine.

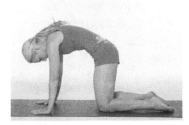

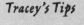

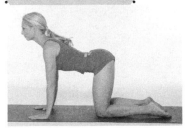

A. Start on your hands and knees. Place your hands shoulder-width apart, directly under your shoulders, and your knees under your hips. Push your chest away from the floor so that you're not sinking in between the shoulder blades and contract the abs.

B. Exhale, draw in the abdominal wall up against the belly button, then tilt the pelvis forward, curling your tailbone under as your spine rounds like that of an angry cat. Then inhale and extend the spine, reaching out through the crown of the head and tailbone while still contracting the abs.

Team Mallett Success Story

Erica Shepherd, 25, Seattle, WA

Lost

21 pounds

3 dress sizes

15 total inches

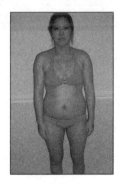 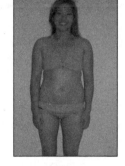

Before   After

• • • • •

Having been active and in shape most of her life, Erica found gaining weight during and after her two pregnancies "depressing and hard to cope with." It didn't help when friends and family would brush off her weight concerns by saying, "You're young. The weight will come off in no time!" "Easier said than done," says Erica. "I still didn't feel good about myself and didn't like how I became totally inactive after being married and having two kids."

All that changed once she joined Team Mallett. Though the Super Fit Mama plan can be divided into small chunks throughout the day, Erica preferred doing them all together. "This works best with my schedule, though I do love having the option of spreading the workouts out if things come up—something that happens often with little ones," says Erica. In just about three weeks, Erica saw big changes. "I was so excited when I went for a jog and to my amazement I lasted A LOT longer than I usually do!" she says. "Before I could barely run a quarter of a mile, but in just about three weeks was able to push a whole mile! I used to always blame my lack of running on my asthma, but just doing the Super Fit Mama strength workouts had increased my cardio strength . . . and I didn't even know it!" Erica's not the only one who noticed these changes. Friends have called her "the Incredible Shrinking Woman." "All my mommy friends want to know how I did it with two small babies and working!" she says.

What she loved about the Super Fit Mama program was that it's "a package deal. You can't work out and not eat right and vice versa." When it came to changing her diet, Erica cleaned all the junk food out of her kitchen. Then she went to the grocery store to stock up on fresh vegetables, lean proteins, and healthy snacks that she pre-portioned so it would be quick and easy for her to grab food on the go. "I also went from eating one to two HUGE meals of high carbs and fat a day to eating small meals every three hours and more fresh vegetables," she says. She also began cooking more often and skipping the drive-thru meals that her family had enjoyed too often in the past.

Of course, sticking to this plan wasn't always easy. "I admit that I thought about throwing in the towel a couple times, but I kept thinking about the big picture. Do I want to be healthier? Do I want to set a good example for my kids? Do I want to look good in that darn bridesmaids dress? Yes, yes, and YES!!" she says. That kind of determination has paid off in more ways than one. Not only is Erica healthier and trimmer, but her self-esteem is soaring. "Since doing the program, I've gained the confidence to finally finish my Pilates certification after a five-year break and just feel happier about my life in general!"

MOTIVATION FROM TEAM MALLETT

"After my first pregnancy, I'd pee a little bit every time I sneezed or coughed. Pilates really helped, but the incontinence returned—and seemed even worse—after my second child was born. It was uncomfortable and embarrassing to leak when I ran or jumped, and the skipping rope segment in my favorite workout DVD sent me to the bathroom every time. This can be a HUGE barrier with getting back into shape because it's hard to have the confidence to work out when you're worried about peeing your pants. I'm happy to say that the ab exercises in the Super Fit Mama plan have definitely helped!"—Andrea Frye

THE BENEFITS OF POSTNATAL EXERCISE

1. It helps to reduce postnatal depression known as the "baby blues."
2. It can help you recover more quickly so you're back to your pre-pregnancy body faster.
3. It provides a much-needed energy boost.
4. It's a great stress release and gives you a little time to focus on yourself.
5. It helps you strengthen your body for the demands of lifting and carrying your baby (and prepare for the days ahead when you're chasing an active toddler).

CHAPTER 7

BODY AFTER BABY PHASE I
7–19 Weeks Postpartum

WITH SIX WEEKS OF MOTHERHOOD UNDER YOUR BELT, you're probably tired and weary. But you may also be even more eager to shed the pregnancy pounds and take those maternity clothes out of your wardrobe rotation. The good news is that by now you've probably gotten the okay from your doctor to resume your pre-pregnancy exercise plan.

But the task ahead shouldn't feel overwhelming, because if you stick with the Super Fit Mama plan you *will* get your body back. It may seem like you've got a huge mountain to climb, and you're probably not sure how you're going to fit exercise in between changing diapers and feeding your baby. I remember looking in the mirror, not recognizing my own body, and worrying: What if I couldn't find the time to work out and couldn't lose the weight? Trust me, once you get that endorphin rush and energetic feeling from working out and eating nutritious foods, you'll want to make the time. It may not be smooth sailing in the beginning, but once you've tasted the good life it's hard to go back to feeling sluggish, emotional, depressed, and frustrated. All it takes is just a few small steps.

Step one: Change your attitude! When I work with clients, I know right away who is going to succeed by their energetic attitude and level of optimism. Now I know it's hard to keep thinking positive 24/7 and that we all have setbacks. But if that happens, just remember that you are not alone. Marley from Team Mallett kept her focus by surrounding herself with upbeat poems and positive affirmations and listening to empowering CDs while she was driving. When I felt frustrated at my uphill battle, I would look at old photos and make a promise to myself to keep up the hard work to get my body back. It's important to get rid of negativity in all areas of your life, not just when it comes to diet and exercise. Of course, it's so easy to put yourself down, and seems strange to give yourself a compliment. But being critical is a waste of energy—and with a new baby, and a body to whip into shape, you don't have an ounce of energy to spare.

So what do you do? Start by countering negative thoughts with positive ones (either in your head or on paper). Instead of, "I'm so tired there's

> For a workout log, go to the Resource section of this book, or download one from my website at www.tracey mallett.com.

absolutely no way I can exercise today," tell yourself, "I'm feeling a little tired today, but I can manage 15 minutes and tomorrow I will try to double it." Replace "I hate my fat thighs" with "My legs and thighs need some work, but I can feel the exercises starting to make a difference," or "Each day, I'm getting closer to my goal." Being positive is the only way to move forward and feel empowered. Do you want your children hearing negative words about your body or exercise (and adopting these attitudes, too)?

Step two: Write an action plan! After all, without a plan on paper there is no plan. Kristina from Team Mallett scheduled her workouts in her Blackberry because it "forced her to exercise." After all, if she deleted these meetings with herself, she said, it was like admitting failure. How you draft your plan is up to you and your personal style. Maybe it works to have a big wipe-off calendar to help plan out your week against your family's schedule. Or maybe you'd prefer to schedule it on your computer or write it out by hand. My point is that all you have to do is pick your days and "just do it." *Saying* you're going to exercise is not enough—especially now that you're a mom with an unpredictable schedule. Ultimately, however you write down your action plan, it comes down to taking action.

Step three: Set a realistic goal! Without a goal, you have no way of measuring your success, and each little success (like a pound lost or a pair of pants that's too big) will be your biggest motivator. That's why I encourage you to take a photo of yourself today so that you can see the changes for yourself as you progress. A camera may be the last thing you want to see right now, but trust me, when you're lean and mean, you'll be thrilled to whip out your "before" photo and see how far you've come. When you set your goals, try dividing them into mini stages. For example, if you need to lose 30 pounds, start with a goal of 10 pounds. If your goal is to be able to run 5 miles, set a goal of 2 miles. This makes them seem more manageable and attainable. To get a clear vision of how you can realistically achieve your goals, answer the following questions before you set them.

1. How long do you think it will take you to reach your goal?
2. What mini goals can you set to get to your ultimate goal?
3. Is your goal realistic? (Be honest with yourself!)
4. What do you need to have at hand to be able to start to reach for your goal?

5. What are the main obstacles that may prevent you from achieving this goal?
6. What actions do you need to take in order to bypass your obstacles?

Step four: Get support! You may feel embarrassed or silly sharing your goals with other people (especially those who never struggled with their weight), but it's so helpful. You're more likely to stick with your healthy exercise and eating plan if you're accountable to someone. Team Mallett found that joining the online group at www.teammallett.com kept them committed. Seeing other women's results inspired them to keep going. Others used weekly blogging as a way to be accountable: Posting their hopes and actions made them more likely to stick to the plan and brought them greater success.

Step five: Lose the guilt! Yes, I know that's much easier said than done and it's something that every mom struggles with. How could we think of taking time for ourselves when we have children who need us? Well, sometimes a little break for your kids not only does you a world of good but is good for them, too. Dropping them off at Grandma's or at the child-care facility at your gym is not such a bad thing. They will interact with other people or children and truly appreciate when they see you in an hour's time, and you will feel better that you have moved your body and released some stress. I like to call it rejuvenation. This makes it a better family environment for everyone, which is why my kids say that "Mommy is much nicer after going to the gym."

Step six: Find the time! I know, I know, it's another one of those things that's easier said than done. But doing so is a must if you're going to reach your goals. The number one excuse not to exercise is "I don't have time to exercise." From now on, I want you to erase that phrase from your mind and remember that finding time is all about prioritizing your schedule. You may have to get up 30 minutes before the baby gets up, break a sweat when the baby is taking a nap, or exercise to a DVD while your little one is mesmerized by a toy. The gals on Team Mallett also had difficulties with the time factor. Some of the women worked full time, while others cared for multiple children—and some did both! However, after a trial period they finally got into a routine, and their success stories are here in the book to inspire you to do the same.

GETTING STARTED

Because I've created the following plan with new moms in mind, it's made up of little chunks of exercise that you can squeeze into your busy, busy life. It also combines both cardio and strength training so that you can torch fat and calories while building lean, long muscles. Talk about multitasking! But before starting the Super Fit Mama plan, you need to do a few things.

1. Take three full-length photos of yourself: one of your front, another of your side, and a third of your back. Wear something that shows some skin, such as a workout bra and shorts.

2. Measure yourself in the following spots: your chest, hips, waist, arms, and thighs. (See sidebar, "How to Measure Correctly," in this chapter.) I recommend remeasuring yourself every three to four weeks or trying on the same few pieces of clothing to see how they fit.

3. Weigh yourself. I know this isn't fun, but this will be your starting weight and what you'll compare yourself to each week as you shed pounds. Weigh yourself every one or two weeks at the same time of day, on the same day of the week, and, importantly, on the same scale.

4. Make a copy of your workout, food journal, and progress sheet from the Resources section of this book, or download it from my website at www.traceymallett.com.

5. Clean out your kitchen and get rid of any high-calorie, nutritionally empty, or highly processed foods. If you feel guilty because you've got kids or a husband who love these snacks, know that they shouldn't be eating this junk either. (There are

HOW TO MEASURE CORRECTLY

- Chest: Place the tape measure around your breasts and in line with your nipples.
- Waist: Measure around your waist in line with your belly button.
- Hips: Measure below the boney part of your hip bones (approximately 3 to 4 inches from your waist). In other words, measure the widest part of your hips, including your butt.
- Arms: Measure around the middle of your upper arm between your shoulder and the elbow. Don't forget to measure both arms.
- Thighs: Measure around the widest part of each thigh.

plenty of healthy—but decadent-tasting—foods that your family will love listed in chapters 10 and 11.)

6. Go shopping and stock the pantry with nutritious foods. Place them at eye level. This will remind you what foods you need to eat for success.

THE BODY AFTER BABY PHASE I WORKOUT PLAN

So how does this plan actually work? Don't worry, I've made it incredibly simple because I remember what life was like with a newborn. All the conditioning workouts are in segments of only 6 to 10 minutes, which gives you some flexibility to fit exercise into your unpredictable schedule. In addition to these segments, I've included workouts for you to do with your baby on the go—the diaper bag workout, stroller burn, and the baby legs workout—exercises you can do with your baby at any time. These can be done for extra calorie burn or on days when you just don't have a minute to yourself. Table 7.1 shows what your schedule should look like. Now I'm a mom, too, so I know that you won't be able to follow it to the letter; do your best, and when it doubt, just move your body!

TABLE 7.1: PHASE I SAMPLE WORKOUT PLAN

WORKOUTS	MONDAY	TUESDAY	WEDNESDAY	THURSDAY	FRIDAY	SATURDAY	SUNDAY
Circuit							
A, B & C	*		*		*		
Lose the Mommy Tummy	*	*	*		*	*	
Mama Butt Blast	*		*	*	*		
Super Flexibility	*		*		*		
Cardio							
20–30 Minutes		*		*		*	

PHASE I POSTPARTUM CARDIO STRENGTH TRAINING CIRCUIT

Time: 6 to 8 minutes per circuit segment.

How to: Perform each exercise once using the recommended set of weights. Repeat if you'd like to do another set. I've suggested a number of reps for each exercise, but if you are just starting out, you may start lower and work up to these targets.

You'll need: Two sets of dumbbells. (For each exercise I've indicated which set of dumbbells to use with the terms "Lighter" and "Heavier." These could be 3-lb. and 5-lb. weights, or, if you're just starting out, you might choose to use 1-lb. and 3-lb. weights instead, or 2-lb. and 4-lb. weights. If one set seems too heavy for you, go with a lighter set until you are ready to move up.)

While performing the exercises in the cardio strength circuits, try and engage the pelvic floor on every exhale.

Warm-up: Walk around the house, march in place, or dance with your baby for a few minutes. This gradually increases your core body temperature and warms up the muscles. Take deep breaths.

CIRCUIT A

1. Plié to lunge with upward row

Muscles targeted: Glutes, hamstrings, quads, calves, shoulders, and biceps

Inspiration: To blast Mommy cellulite

Reps: 15 in each position

Weights: Lighter

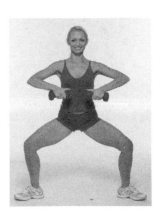 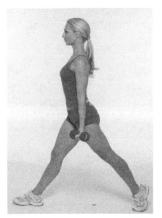 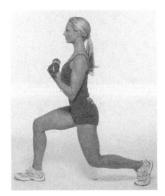

A. Start with your legs shoulder-width apart, knees and toes pointing to the corners of the room, legs turned out at the hips. The arms are straight in front of the torso and your palms are facing toward your body. Bend your knees over your toes into a plié position as you bend your elbows, drawing your hands toward your chest in an upright row. Lower the arms as you straighten your legs and turn to the left side.

B. Perform a lunge with your hips facing to the left as you bicep curl the arms. Extend the legs and return back to the plié position and upright row. Repeat the sequence 15 times, then switch to the other side.

Tracey's Tips

Always keep your knees over the first and second toe in both plié and lunge. When performing an upright row, try not to elevate your shoulders, which may cause stress in your neck and shoulders.

2. Lunge to overhead press (starting in bicep hammer curl)

Muscles targeted: Glutes, hamstrings, quads, calves, biceps, and shoulders

Inspiration: Burn total body fat in one move!

Reps: 12

Weights: Lighter

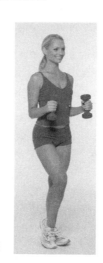

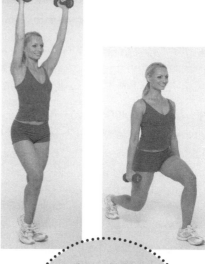

A. Stand tall with your right foot resting on the ball of your foot and your arms bent by your sides. Lift your arms overhead with palms facing inward and then bring them down through a bicep curl.

B. Step back with your right foot into a lunge with your hips facing forward as you extend your arms. Next, bring your right leg and your arms back to the start position. Do 12 reps, then switch legs and do 12 more.

Note: Place weights on the floor.

Tracey's Tips

As you step back, keep your knee over your toes and only bend as far as feels comfortable; go no lower than a 90-degree angle.

Cardio

Knee twist rotation for 60 seconds.

Muscles targeted: Legs and obliques

Inspiration: Muffin top blaster!

Start with your arms overhead and then lift your right leg toward your chest as you bend your arms and twist your upper body toward the knee. Focus on working your obliques as you twist your body. Alternate legs and twist to the other side. Repeat for 60 seconds.

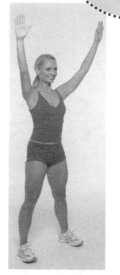

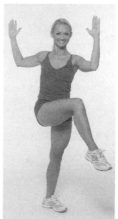

3. Chair or coffee table push-ups with leg extensions

Muscles targeted: Chest, arms, abs, glutes, and hamstrings

Inspiration: Sexy sculpted arms!

Reps: 10 with each leg extended for a total of 20 reps

A. Place your hands on the corners of a coffee table or chair, shoulder-width apart, with your legs extended behind you in a push-up position. Lift your right leg off the floor to hip height.

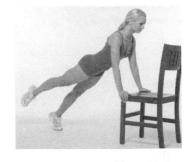

B. Inhale as you bend your elbows toward the chair or coffee table and exhale as you draw your abs toward the spine and straighten the elbows. Do 10 reps with your right leg lifted, then 10 with the left leg lifted.

4. Overhead punching

Muscles targeted: Mid to upper back, posterior deltoids (shoulders), and legs

Inspiration: Time to stop slouching!

Reps: 16

Weights: Lighter

Tracey's Tips

Only go down as far as you can without moving your shoulder blades or sagging in between them. Imagine you're pushing away from the floor, activating the lats and stabilizing the upper shoulder girdle. Focus on pulling your abs in so that you protect the lower back.

Tracey's Tips

Be careful not to over-arch the back. Draw your abdominals toward the spine and pull your shoulders down toward your hips.

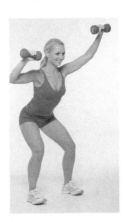
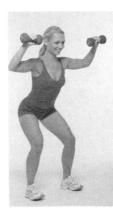

A. Start with the legs shoulder-width apart in a deep squat position and pitch your torso slightly forward from your hips, with your elbows bent and your hands level with your shoulders.

B. Extend your right arm overhead, and as you bring it back to the start position, reach the opposite hand overhead. Stay low in the squat to work the legs.

Note: Place weights on the floor.

Cardio:

Repeat knee twist rotation for 60 seconds.

CIRCUIT B

1. Small plié squat with shoulder raise and angled bicep curls

Muscles targeted: Quads, glutes, shoulders, and biceps

Inspiration: No more lower body flab and jiggly arms!

Reps: 10 on each leg

Weights: Lighter

A. Stand with your legs turned out at the hips and your right knee bent, with your foot resting on a toe in a small "V" position. Place your arms by your sides with the palms facing upward.

B. Next, perform a bicep curl with the arms angled on a slight diagonal for a total of 10 reps with 10 small pulses, then switch legs and repeat.

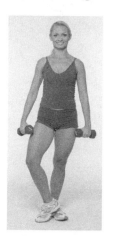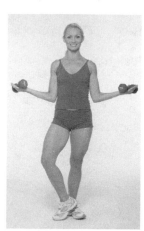

Tracey's Tips

Do not overarch the lower back. Remember to draw your tailbone under and pull in your abdominals, and do your Kegels as you exhale!

2. Plié squat with shoulder circles

Muscles targeted: Quads, hamstrings, glutes, and shoulders

Inspiration: To be able to pick up your baby with ease

Reps: 8 in each direction

Weights: Lighter

Tracey's Tips

Keep all the movements just a little lower than the shoulders and never bring arms above the shoulders.

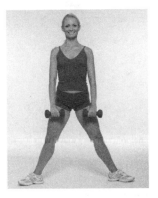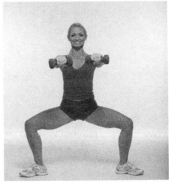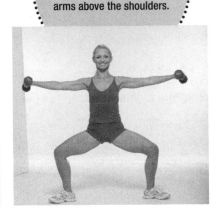

A. Start with your legs shoulder-width apart, turned out at the hips, and your toes pointed out to the corners of the room. Rest your hands on your thighs.

Note: Place weights on the floor.

B. Bend your legs with the knees going over the toes and lift the arms straight forward to shoulder height. Extend the legs, take the arms out to your sides, and then return them back to the start position. Repeat for 8 reps, then reverse the arm circles.

Cardio:

Jump twist for 60 seconds.

Muscles targeted: Arms and legs

Inspiration: Shrink your waist!

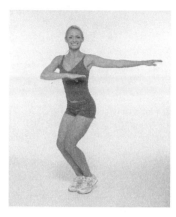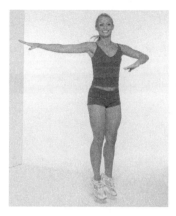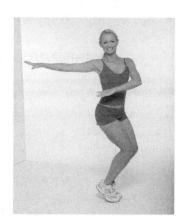

Start with the feet together, balancing on the balls of your feet, and your knees twisted to the right side. Place both arms at shoulder height toward the left side of the body. At a moderate pace, do small jumps, twisting the legs and arms in opposite directions.

Modification: If you have knee or back issues, then do not jump; always keep one foot on the floor.

3. Plié with rotation

Muscles targeted: Quads, hamstrings, glutes, triceps, and obliques

Inspiration: To stand taller and feel confident again!

Reps: 30

Weights: Lighter

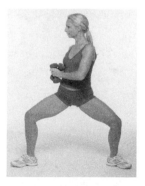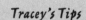

Tracey's Tips

Try to keep the pelvis and lower body as still as possible. This will make you use the muscles of your waist— called the obliques—more effectively.

A. Start with your feet a little further than shoulder-width apart, with your toes pointing to the corners of the room and your legs turned out at the hips. Bend both knees and hold onto the dumbbells in front of your torso.

B. Exhale and twist the body to the right side, then the left, keeping the pelvis facing forward and the knees bent in a plié position. Perform 30 reps, with a twist to both right and left counting as one rep.

4. Row with external rotation

Muscles targeted: Mid to upper back and rotator cuff

Inspiration: Say goodbye to shoulder pain. It worked for me!

Reps: 10

Weights: Lighter

Note: Place weights on the floor.

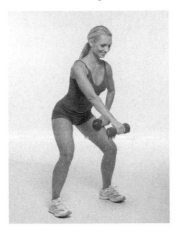 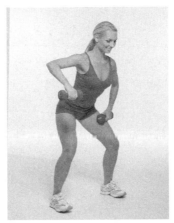 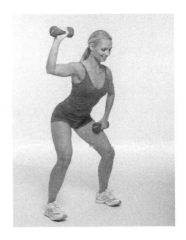

A. Start with your feet shoulder-width apart and your knees bent in a squat with your torso slightly pitched forward from the waist. Place your left hand on your thigh and reach your right arm forward at chest height, palm facing downward.

B. Inhale as you bend your right elbow back to the side of your body, squeezing your right shoulder blade toward the middle of the back. Exhale and rotate the forearms up so that your palms are facing forward and your elbow is directly under your wrist. Do 10 reps on the right, then 10 on the left.

Tracey's Tips

Keep your hand and elbow in line as you draw the shoulder blade toward the center of your spine. Keep the shoulder blades down as you rotate the forearms. Always draw you abs toward the spine so that you don't overarch the lower back.

CIRCUIT C

1. Step plié to side (2 to each side) with shoulder raise

Muscles targeted: Glutes, quads, hamstrings, and arms

Inspiration: Beautiful toned arms and a nice perky butt!

Reps: 6 to each direction

Weights: Lighter

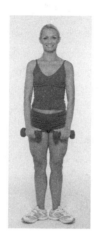 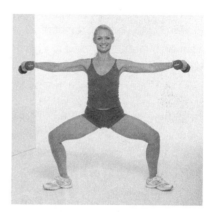

A. Start with your legs turned out at the hips and your feet in a small "V" position, arms at your sides.

B. Step out to the right and bend your knees into a plié position while at the same time you extend your arms out to the sides, shoulder height, leading with the elbows. Draw your left foot toward your right foot, pulling the inner thighs together and returning to a small "V" position. Repeat one more time to the right side and then move in the other direction.

Modification: If your shoulders get tired and you start feeling stress in the neck, then give your arms a break and just continue with the legs.

Cardio:

Repeat jump twist for 60 seconds.

> **Tracey's Tips**
>
> Imagine that you're zipping the inner thighs together as you pull the heels together. Draw your abs in toward the spine and keep your spine in a neutral position. Be careful not to overarch the spine in the plié position.

2. Lunge with bent-over row

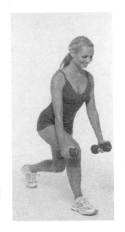
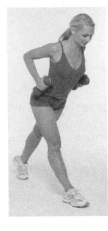

Muscles targeted: Mid to upper back, quads, hamstrings, and glutes

Inspiration: Four words: no more back fat!!

Reps: 15 on each side

Weights: Heavier

A. Start with your right leg in front of you, toes pointing forward, and your left leg behind you, resting on a toe. Your hips are facing forward and both knees are bent. Now pitch your torso forward from the hips and bring your arms forward, level with your shoulders, palms facing toward each other.

B. Exhale and extend the front knee, drawing your shoulder blades together as you bring your elbows behind your body in a bent-over row. Inhale and bend the knees as you extend your elbows, then repeat.

Note: Place weights on the floor.

Tracey's Tips

Keep your knees over the toes as you bend your front knee and keep the abs tight so that you don't overarch the back. Focus on drawing the shoulder blades down the back and squeezing them to-gether.

Cardio:

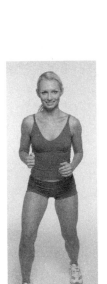
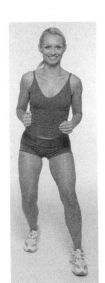
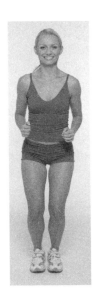

"Out, Out, In, In," for 60 seconds.

Muscles targeted: Legs

Inspiration: Athletic, toned legs!

Start with the legs together, hands bent in front of the chest. Step out to the right then out to the left (steps should be about hip-width apart). Then bring the right leg back in to start, followed by the left leg. Continue going out, out, in, in, as fast as you can manage.

3. Windmill rotation

Muscles targeted: Quads, hamstrings, glutes, arms, mid to upper back, and obliques

Inspiration: A tiny waist and a sculpted back!

Reps: 10 on each side

Weights: Lighter

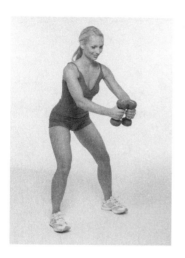 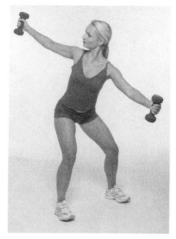 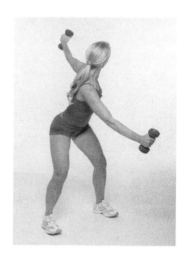

A. Start with your legs shoulder-width apart, toes pointing forward and knees bent in a squat position. Extend your arms forward at shoulder height with palms facing each other.

B. Exhale and rotate the torso as you reach the right arm out and around toward the back right-hand corner with your gaze following the hand. Inhale and return back to the front. Repeat on the other side, then continue, alternating sides while staying in a static squat position.

Tracey's Tips

Keep your hips facing forward as you rotate the torso, and be careful not to elevate the shoulder. Draw the shoulder blade down and back toward the pelvis.

4. Rotator cuff with biceps in plié position

Muscles targeted: Shoulders, rotator cuff, biceps, quads, hamstrings, and glutes

Inspiration: Beautiful sculpted shoulders and a nice round butt!

Reps: 15–20

Weights: Lighter

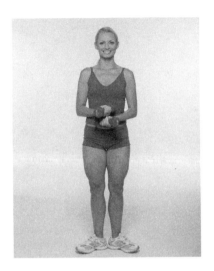 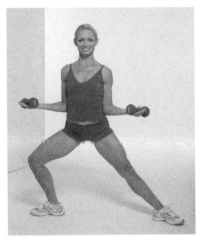

A. Start with the legs turned out at the hips and your feet in a small "V" position, elbows bent close to your body and forearms crossed in front of your torso with the palms facing upward.

B. Step out to the right side and bend the right knee as you open the arms to the side, keeping the elbows close to the body. Draw the right leg back to the start position as you cross the forearms in front of the chest, and then repeat to the other side as you alternate the legs.

Note: Place weights on the floor.

Cardio:

Repeat "Out, Out, In, In," for 60 seconds.

Cooldown: Walk in place. Start with your arms moving in a circular pattern as you walk in place. The circles gradually get smaller as your heart rate slowly comes down.

Tracey's Tips

Keep the elbows glued to the sides of your body. To really work those glutes and legs, go a little deeper into the plié and—oh baby—feel the burn!

PHASE I LOSE YOUR MOMMY TUMMY BLAST

The following exercises can be performed after you have your doctor's clearance to exercise. Also, be sure to continue with the post-pregnancy exercises described in Chapter 6, as these are your foundation for getting your tummy back in shape. If you're starting the plan at this stage, please familiarize yourself with the Chapter 6 exercises before you start to add the Phase I Lose Your Mommy Tummy section. If you still have an abdominal separation (diastasis recti), look for the star next to some of the following exercises so you know which ones are safe to perform at this stage.

Time: 6 to 8 minutes.

How to: Perform each exercise for one set.

You'll need: A rolled-up towel or exercise band and a pillow.

1. Pelvic bridges with figure eights*

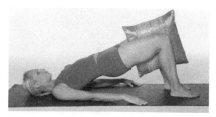

Reps: 5 each direction

A. Place a pillow between your knees and lie on your back with your knees bent and your feet hip-width apart. Your heels are in line with your sit bones, and your hands are by your sides.

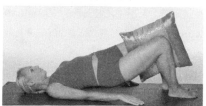

B. Exhale as you draw in your abs and do a pelvic tilt, rolling up through the spine until you're in a bridge position.

C. Tilt the pelvis toward the right side and move up and around, making a sideways figure eight. (The middle of the eight is the starting bridge position.) After performing five in each direction, slowly roll down through the spine, breathing space in between each vertebra until you're lying on your back in a neutral spine position.

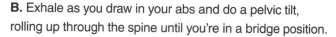

Tracey's Tips

Focus on squeezing the pillow and drawing up your pelvic floor throughout the figure eight.

2. Abs towel pulse

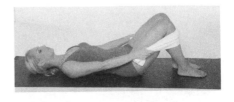

Reps: 10–20

A. Lie on your back with your knees and heels in line with your sit bones. Wrap a towel around your knees and hold onto the ends of it at the sides of your thighs as you squeeze your inner thighs together.

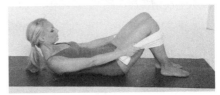

Tracey's Tips

Your focus should always be on pulling in the abdominal wall, not pushing it out. Try and add a "Quick Flick" Kegel with every exhale (see Chapter 2).

Every time you resist the towel, exhale and draw the abs in toward the spine. This will make your abs work harder.

B. Exhale, drawing in the abdominals as you lift your head, neck, and shoulders off the floor. Hold this position as you perform 10–12 tiny up-and-down pulses, then roll back down.

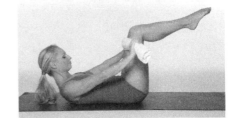

3. Towel-resisted single-leg stretch

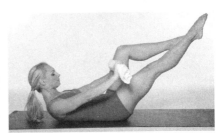

Reps: 10 on each leg

A. Lie on your back with your knees directly above your hips, knees bent at a 90-degree angle and shins parallel to the floor. Place the rolled-up towel in front of your thighs with your hands holding onto each end to create resistance. Contract the abs as you pull your knees toward your chest and push the towel in the opposite direction. Lift your head, neck, and shoulders off the floor.

B. Extend the right leg out, still resisting with the opposite knee, and exhale. Then switch legs and repeat to the other side.

Modification: Keep your head on the floor.

4. Heel reach

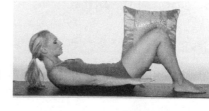

Reps: 10 on each side

A. Place a pillow between your legs and lie on your back with your feet hip-width apart, heels in line with your sit bones and hands by your sides.

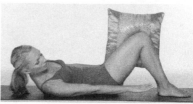

B. Lift your head, neck, and shoulders off the floor. Exhale and reach your right hand toward the right heel as you bend your right side. Inhale, return to center, then repeat to the other side. Keep your head off the floor throughout the exercise.

Tracey's Tips

Imagine that your lowest rib and hip bone are moving together as you side bend, and look toward the heel that you're reaching for.

5. Chest lift with single-leg lift and rotation

Reps: 10 on each leg without rotation, and 10 on each leg with rotation

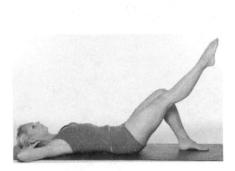 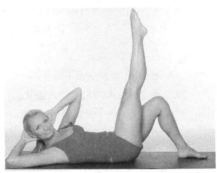

A. Lie on your back with your right leg bent, heel in line with your right sit bone, and your left leg extended level with the right knee. Hands behind the head.

D. Exhale, lift the head, neck, and shoulders off the floor, and at the same time lift the right leg toward the chest. Repeat, alternating knees for 10 reps on each leg. Next, rotate the left shoulder to the right leg and the right shoulder to the left knee as you continue alternating legs.

Modification: Bend the working leg into a 45-degree angle.

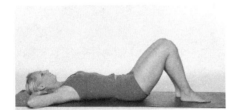 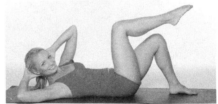

Tracey's Tips

Keep your elbows still, and move from your torso, not your shoulders, for a true rotation. Look toward the direction you're traveling in order to get more rotation and work the oblique muscles more effectively.

6. Lower abs curl tilt

Reps: 10

A. Place a pillow between your inner thighs and lie on your back with your hands by your sides. Your legs are slightly bent and extended up to the ceiling.

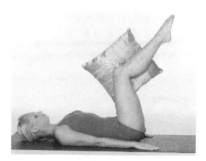

B. Exhale and curl the pelvis, drawing your pubic bone up to your belly button into a pelvic tilt. Limit the movement of the legs as they reach straight up to the ceiling (not toward the face). Inhale and lower the tailbone gently onto the mat, then repeat.

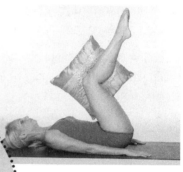

*Modification: If you have diastasis recti, perform a pelvic tilt with one leg lifted and the other leg bent at the knee with the foot resting on the floor.

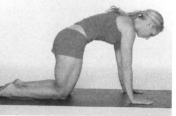

Tracey's Tips

The movement will be very small at first until you build strength in your lower abdominals, but keep trying because you *will* see progress if you're persistent.

Keep your upper body stable and don't sink in between the shoulder blades.

7. Wag the tail 1*

Reps: 10 to each side

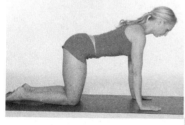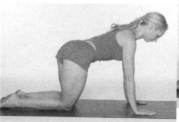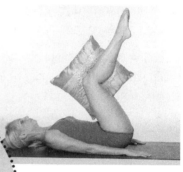

A. Position yourself on your hands and knees. Make sure your hands are shoulder-width apart and directly under your shoulders and your knees are stacked under your hips.

B. Move your hips to the right as if you were a dog wagging your tail, and then draw your abs in and do a pelvic tilt. Return back to center, then repeat to the other side.

8. Side plank lifts*

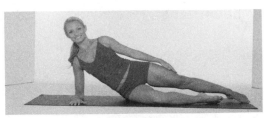

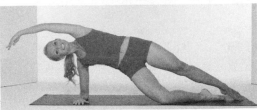

Reps: 10 on each side

A. Start by sitting on your right hip with your right leg slightly bent and your left leg extended straight out to the side. Balance on your right forearm with your elbow bent. Make sure your elbow is directly underneath your shoulder. You should be drawing your shoulder blade down toward your hips, which helps release stress in the upper body.

B. Exhale as you lift your hips off the floor and reach your left arm up and over into a side stretch. Hold and then gently lower down. Repeat 10 times before going to the other side.

Modifications: Keep both knees bent.

With every exhale and rep of each exercise, try and perform a Kegel. This will intensify the abdominal contraction and help you get your much-needed quota of Kegels in for the day.

Tracey's Tips

Keep your hips stacked and facing forward throughout the exercise and draw your shoulders away from your ears. Always place your elbow directly under your shoulder joint.

PHASE I MAMA BUTT BLAST

Time: 6 to 8 minutes.

How to: Perform one set of each exercise.

You'll need: Light to medium-intensity exercise band (The exercises can be done without the exercise band if you prefer.).

Note: All of the following exercises are safe to perform with a diastasis recti.

1. Step side grand pliés

Muscles targeted: Glutes, quads, and hamstrings

Inspiration: Get rid of thigh wobble fast!

Reps: 8 on each side

A. Wrap your band tightly around your calves and tie it in front. Turn your legs out at the hips and stand with your feet in a small "V" position (ballet first position). Extend your arms out to the sides, slightly rounded at shoulder height.

B. Step your right foot out to the side a little further than shoulder-width apart into a plié position, with your knees over your toes, then bend your knees into a deep plié (or as far as you feel comfortable). Extend your arms out to the side at shoulder height, slightly rounded. Then bring the right leg and arms back to the starting position as you straighten the legs. Do 8 reps, then switch legs and repeat on the other side.

> **Tracey's Tips**
>
> Try doing the exercise without the band first to get familiar with the move, then add the band. Keep the band taut at all times to most effectively work the lower body muscles.

Modification: Perform without the band. If balance is an issue, hold onto a chair for support or plié without the transfer back to a "V" position.

2. Donkey kick

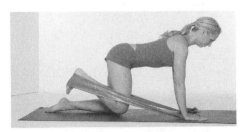

Muscles targeted: Glutes, hamstrings, and quads

Inspiration: To make pregnancy-induced cellulite a thing of the past!

Reps: 10 extensions and 10 pulses on each side

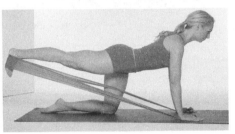

A. Start by kneeling on all fours with your hands directly under the shoulders and your knees directly under your hips. Wrap the exercise band around your right foot and hold the ends of the band in your hands. Lift the right knee about 8 inches off the floor, flexing your foot.

B. Push your heel out behind you as you extend the leg to hip height. Do 10–15 reps, then hold the leg at hip height and pulse up and down for 10–15 reps. Lower the leg and repeat to the other side.

Modification: Perform without the band.

Tracey's Tips

Keep the hips stable by drawing in your abs, and try not to sink in between your shoulder blades.

Keep the knee and shin parallel to the floor and the hips stacked, facing forward. Lift your upper body up and out of the floor and try not to sink in the shoulders.

3. Side kick with pulses

Muscles targeted: Glutes, quads, and hamstrings

Inspiration: No more maternity pants!

Reps: 10–15 on each leg with 10 pulses

A. Lie on your right hip with your right elbow bent, balancing on the forearm. Wrap the band around the left foot, holding the ends of the band in front of your chest on the floor, and bend your knees slightly with the left leg at hip height.

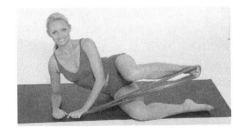

B. Extend the left leg, leading with the heel. Be sure to keep your knee in line with the hip. Do 10–15 reps, then perform tiny pulses (small up and down movements). Repeat the sequence to the other side.

Modification: Perform without the band.

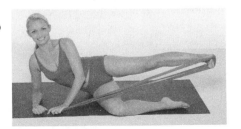

4. Glute blasters!

Muscles targeted: Glutes

Inspiration: A perky dancer's butt!

Reps: 10–15

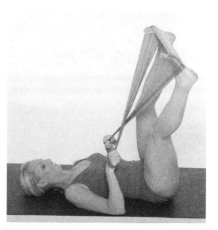

A. Lie on your back with your legs extended up to the ceiling and your toes slightly turned in toward each other. Wrap the band around both feet, cross it in front of your legs, and hold onto the ends in front of your chest. Your elbows are resting on the floor on either side of your torso.

B. Leading with the heels, slightly open the legs a little further than hip-width apart and then return to the start position.

Tracey's Tips

Make the movements small in order to keep the focus on the glutes, and make sure the band stays taut to provide resistance.

Keep the legs as straight as possible, and extend them from the hips, not the knees.

5. Swimming

Muscles targeted: Upper and lower spine, glutes, hamstrings, and obliques

Inspiration: Total rear-view shape-up!

Reps: 10–20 on each side

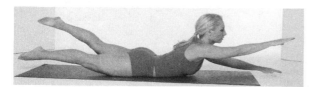

A. Lie on your front with your upper body extended off the floor and your arms extended over your head level with your ears. Lift the legs as you press the pubic bone to the floor.

B. Lift your right arm and left leg a few inches further away from the floor, then switch to the left arm and leg. Alternate at a brisk pace, keeping the torso and head in line with the spine.

6. Heel beats

Muscles targeted: Glutes, inner thighs, and hamstrings

Inspiration: A lifted butt!

Reps: 20

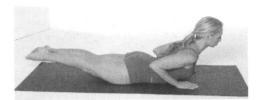 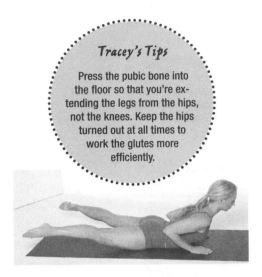

A. Lie on your front with your elbows bent, hands by the sides of your ribcage and legs turned out at the hip so that your heels are together in a small "V" position.

B. Extend the upper body and legs off the floor. Open and close the legs to no further than hip-width apart, beating the heels together at a brisk tempo.

SUPER FIT MAMA FLEXIBILITY

Time: About 6 minutes.

How to: Perform each stretch for 30 seconds, and don't forget to breathe.

1. Pliés, side angle pose

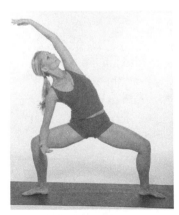

Muscles targeted: Hamstrings, inner thighs, lats, and obliques

Hold for 30 seconds

A. Start with both legs turned out at the hips, toes pointing to the corners of the room and feet shoulder-width apart, and bend the knees over the toes.

B. Rest your right forearm on your right thigh, then lift your left arm up and over toward the right side as you spiral your chest up to the sky. Hold for 30 seconds, then repeat to the other side.

2. Downward dog with walking

Muscles targeted: Hamstrings, calves, and lower, mid, and upper back

Hold for 30 seconds

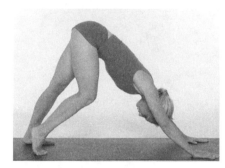

A. Position your hands shoulder-width apart on the floor with your hips extended up to the sky and your feet on the floor, hip-width apart. Your body will form an inverted "V" position.

B. Bend the right knee as you press the left heel into the floor, pause, and then switch legs, holding each stretch for 30 seconds.

3. Kneeling hip flexor stretch

Muscles targeted: Hip flexors and quads

Hold for 30 seconds

Tracey's Tips

Draw in your abs and press the pelvis forward to decrease the arch in the lower back and stretch the hip flexors out.

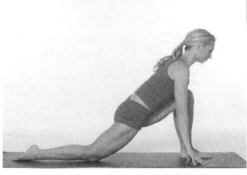

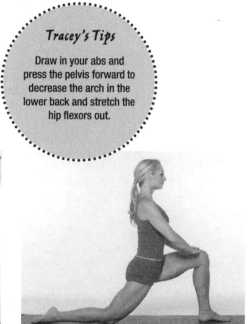

A. Start in a lunge with your back knee resting on the floor and your shin up against a wall. Rest your hands on your knee, straighten your spine, and hold for 30 seconds. Repeat to the other side.

Modifications: Place your hands on either side of your foot. To decrease the amount of stretch, take the knee further away from the wall.

4. Straddle and side stretch

Muscles targeted: Hamstrings, inner thighs, and obliques

Hold each side for 30 seconds

A. Start by sitting on the floor with your legs angled out to the sides. Open them out to a point where you are getting a comfortable stretch. Bend your right elbow and place your right forearm on your right thigh.

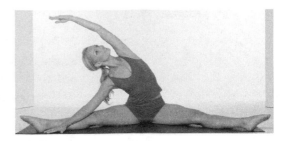

B. Inhale and then exhale as you reach with your left arm up and over to the right side as your torso bends toward the right. Hold for 30 seconds, then repeat to other side.

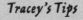

Tracey's Tips

Keep your knees and toes pointing toward the ceiling and try not to roll them forward

Aim to have your hips square to the floor.

5. Pigeon pose

Muscles targeted: Glutes

Hold for 30 seconds on each side

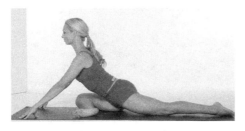

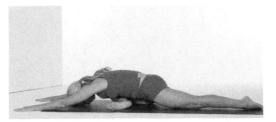

A. Sit on the floor with your right leg in front of you, turned out at the hip with your knee bent at a 45-degree angle, and your left leg extended straight out behind you. Your hips are square, facing forward. This is a common yoga pose.

B. Place your hands on the floor and gently walk them forward to a comfortable position. Hold for 30 seconds, then repeat to the other side.

Modification: Perform the "Sitting glute stretch on the floor" from Chapter 3.

6. Seated spinal rotation

Muscles targeted: Lower back, glutes, and obliques

Hold for 30 seconds on each side

A. Sit tall with your right leg extended forward. Bend your left leg and cross it over your right leg, keeping your hips facing forward.

B. Place your right arm on your left thigh with your fingertips reaching down to the floor. Your left arm is resting on the floor

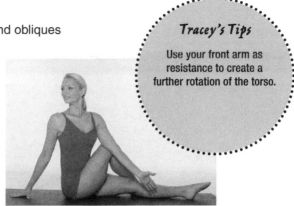

Tracey's Tips

Use your front arm as resistance to create a further rotation of the torso.

slightly behind your left hip as you rotate the torso toward the left, looking toward the back wall. Hold the stretch for 30 seconds, then switch legs and repeat to the other side.

CIRCUIT A

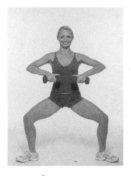
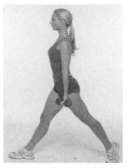
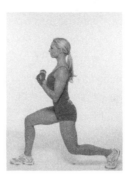

1. PLIÉ TO LUNGE WITH UPWARD ROW

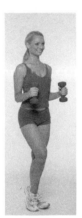
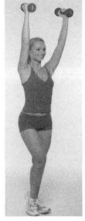
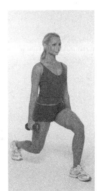

2. LUNGE TO OVERHEAD PRESS (STARTING IN BICEP HAMMER CURL)

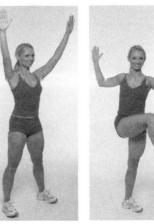

CARDIO: KNEE TWIST ROTATION FOR 60 SECONDS

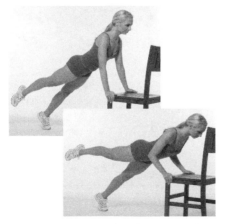
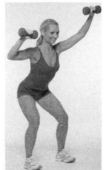
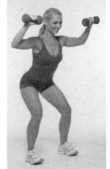

4. OVERHEAD PUNCHING

CARDIO: REPEAT KNEE TWIST ROTATION FOR 60 SECONDS

3. CHAIR OR COFFEE TABLE PUSH-UPS WITH LEG EXTENSIONS

CIRCUIT B

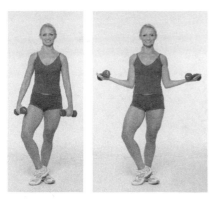

1. ANGLED BICEP CURLS

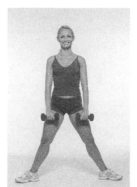 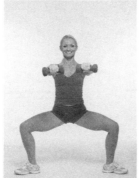 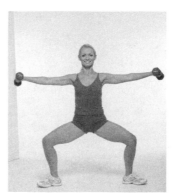

2. PLIÉ SQUAT WITH SHOULDER CIRCLES

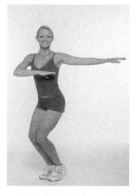 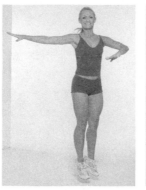 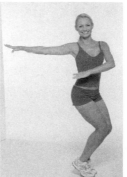

CARDIO: JUMP TWIST FOR 60 SECONDS

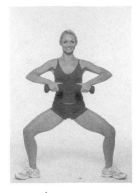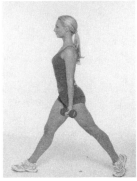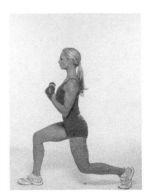

3. PLIÉ WITH ROTATION

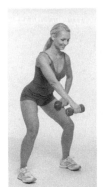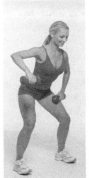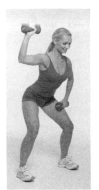

4. ROW WITH EXTERNAL ROTATION

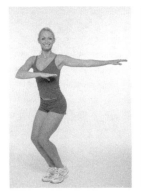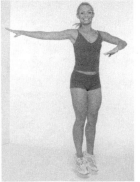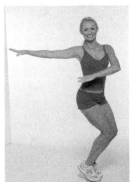

CARDIO: REPEAT JUMP TWIST FOR 60 SECONDS

CIRCUIT C

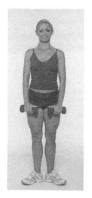 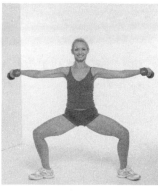

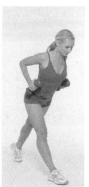
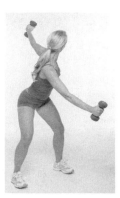

1. STEP PLIÉ TO SIDE (2 TO EACH SIDE) WITH SHOULDER RAISE

2. LUNGE WITH BENT-OVER ROW

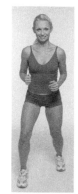 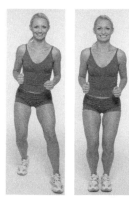

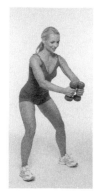 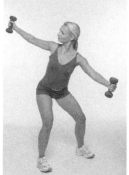

CARDIO: "OUT, OUT, IN, IN," FOR 60 SECONDS

3. WINDMILL ROTATION

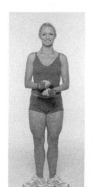 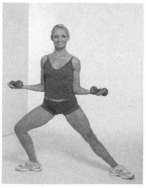

4. ROTATOR CUFF WITH BICEPS IN PLIÉ POSITION

CARDIO: "OUT, OUT, IN, IN," FOR 60 SECONDS

LOSE YOUR MOMMY TUMMY BLAST

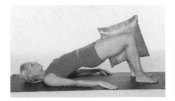 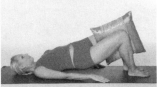 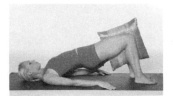

1. PELVIC BRIDGES WITH FIGURE EIGHTS*

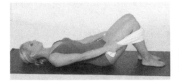 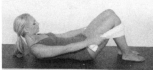

2. ABS TOWEL PULSE

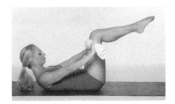 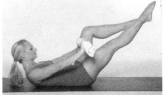

3. TOWEL-RESISTED SINGLE-LEG STRETCH

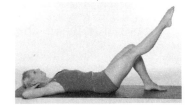

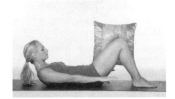 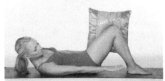

4. HEEL REACH

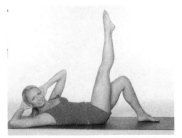

5. CHEST LIFT WITH SINGLE-KNEE LIFT AND ROTATION

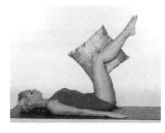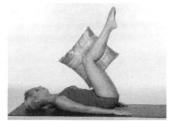

6. LOWER ABS CURL TILT

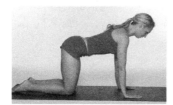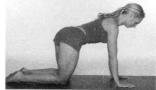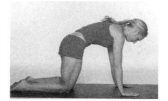

7. WAG THE TAIL 1*

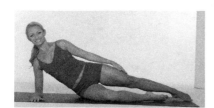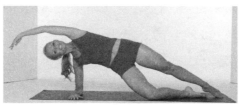

8. SIDE PLANK LIFTS*

MAMA BUTT BLAST

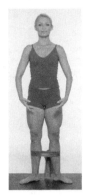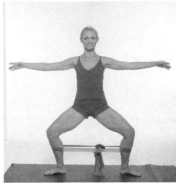

1. STEP SIDE GRAND PLIÉS

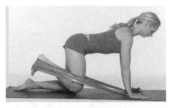
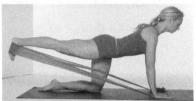

2. DONKEY KICK

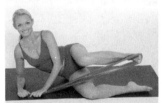
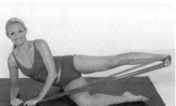
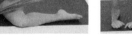

3. SIDE KICK WITH PULSES

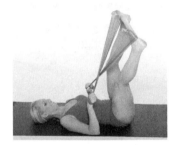

4. GLUTE BLASTERS

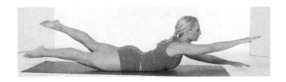

5. SWIMMING

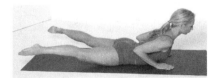
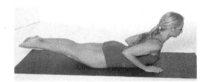

6. HEEL BEATS

SUPER FIT MAMA FLEXIBILITY

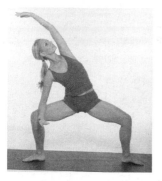

1. PLIÉS, SIDE ANGLE POSE

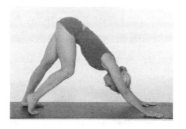

2. DOWNWARD DOG WITH WALKING

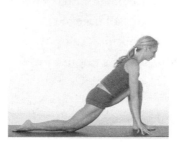

3. KNEELING HIP FLEXOR STRETCH

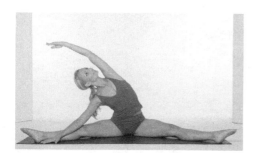

4. STRADDLE AND SIDE STRETCH

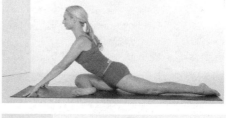

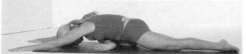

5. PIGEON POSE

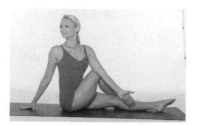

6. SEATED SPINAL ROTATION

CARDIO TIME

By seven weeks' postpartum, I was absolutely dying to do some cardio. I love the endorphin rush and stress relief I get from a good sweat session and was eager to slip on my running shoes. Plus, like you, I really wanted to melt off those pregnancy pounds. However, I learned the hard way that you have to start out at a moderate pace and not overdo it. (As I mentioned in an earlier chapter, I hurt my foot when I did too much too soon and had to hold off on cardio exercise even longer!) You may also think that you can simply pick up where you left off over ten months ago. But even if you were very fit pre-pregnancy, that's not a good idea. You need to give your body a short period of time to rebuild strength and endurance. Don't worry: You're still burning calories, probably more than you would expect because your body is not used to working at this capacity anymore.

INTRODUCTION TO GETTING BACK INTO CARDIO

Here is a plan you can follow for a 30-minute session of walking and light jogging. For the numbers in the last column and what they mean, see the sidebar on "Rate of Perceived Exertion."

Minutes	Activity	Miles per Hour	Rate of Perceived Exertion
0.00–7.00	Walk	3.5–4.5	4
7.00–17.00	Light jog	5.5–6.0	5–6
17.00–22.00	Brisk walk	4.5	4
22.00–27.00	Light jog	5.5–6.0	5–6
27.00–30.00	Walk	3.5	3–4

Note: See Chapter 8 for more on-the-go workouts.

As you get stronger, reduce your walking and increase your running time so that by the end of Phase I you're jogging at a moderate pace for the whole duration. If running does not feel good at this point, then just walk, but increase the intensity by walking faster and climbing inclines for more challenge. When you get to the point that your cardio workout is getting easier, it may be time to try interval workouts. See Chapter 9 for interval workouts.

YOUR REALISTIC GOAL WEIGHT

Your ideal weight depends on several factors: your height, your body type, your muscular build, and your bone structure. Here's how to set a realistic target:

- **Tool One:** First do a simple calculation. Start with 100 pounds for the first five feet of your height, then add an extra 5 pounds for every additional inch. Finally, add a 10-pound buffer on each side of this number. For example, if you're 5 feet 4 inches, your guide weight is 120; with your buffer of 10 pounds, you have a range of 110–130.

RATE OF PERCEIVED EXERTION

Sometimes it's hard to know if you're working hard enough. Though a great way to figure this out is with a heart rate monitor, there's an easy low-tech way to make sure you're pushing yourself hard enough, but not too much. It's a combination of the Rate of Perceived Exertion (RPE) and the talk test.

The talk test is perfect for those of you who are new to exercise or have a pulmonary condition such as asthma. When doing your cardio workouts or segments, you should be able to breathe comfortably, regardless of the intensity. You know that you're overdoing it if you're unable to count or put words together to make sentences. For those of you who have been exercising for a while, the RPE scale is a good tool to use to gauge your efforts. Here's what the numbers will tell you as you're working out. It may seem a bit confusing at first, but with time and practice you'll be able to get a sense of your effort with ease.

RPE 1–2: Very easy. You can talk without any effort.
RPE 3: Easy. You can talk with almost no effort.
RPE 4: Moderately easy. You can talk comfortably without effort.
RPE 5: Moderate. Requires some effort to talk.
RPE 6: Moderately hard. Requires a bit more effort to talk.
RPE 7: Difficult. Requires a lot of effort to talk.
RPE 8: Very difficult. Requires maximum effort to talk.
RPE 9–10: Maximum effort. No talking.

A good sports bra is a must-have item as you venture into the world of post-pregnancy. After all, it's likely that your breasts are bigger than they've ever been—especially if you're breastfeeding—and a lack of support can be very painful and hinder your progress. Lucky for you, there are tons of wonderful sports bras out there, and if you can't find the support you want, simply wear two. (Your best bet is to try and breastfeed before exercising in order to empty your breasts as much as possible to lessen the pain.) Look for bras with wide supportive and adjustable straps. Team Mallett tried and tested the following brands and gave them high marks: Champion Power Sleek Sports Bra (www.championusa.com) and Enell Sport Bra (www.enell.com).

- **Tool Two:** Body Mass Index (BMI) charts estimate your body fat based on your height and weight. They can give you a ballpark figure to see where you currently stand with your body fat percentage and help you decide where you want your healthy weight range to be. However, they do not always provide an accurate BMI figure for women who have a lot of muscle mass. For a more accurate estimate, you would have to get tested; some fitness centers provide this service. (See "Determining Your Body Mass Index" below.)
- **Tool Three:** The clothes test is one of my favorite tools because it feels so liberating when, after months of exercise and a good diet, you can finally fit into your pre-pregnancy pants. We all have our favorite pieces of clothing that we want to get back into, and what better inspiration than hanging them in your closet in clear view?

TABLE 7.2: RISK OF ASSOCIATED DISEASE ACCORDING TO BMI AND WAIST SIZE

BMI	WEIGHT	WAIST LESS THAN OR EQUAL TO 40 INCHES (MEN) OR 35 INCHES (WOMEN)	WAIST GREATER THAN 40 INCHES (MEN) OR 35 INCHES (WOMEN)
18.5 or less	Underweight	N/A	N/A
18.5–24.9	Normal	N/A	N/A
25.0–29.9	Overweight	Increased	High
30.0–34.9	Obese	High	Very high
35.0–39.9	Obese	Very high	Very high
40 or greater	Extremely obese	Extremely high	Extremely high

DETERMINING YOUR BODY MASS INDEX (BMI)

To use the Body Mass Index table to find an estimate of your BMI, find your height in the left-hand column. Move across the row to find your current weight. The number at the top of the column is the BMI for that height and weight and represents the percentage of body fat.

TABLE 7.3: BMI ESTIMATES BY HEIGHT AND WEIGHT

BMI	19	20	21	22	23	24	25	26	27	28	29	30	35	40
HEIGHT (INCHES)	WEIGHT (POUNDS)													
58	91	96	100	105	110	115	119	124	129	134	138	143	167	191
59	94	99	104	109	114	119	124	128	133	138	143	148	173	198
60	97	102	107	112	118	123	128	133	138	143	148	153	179	20
61	100	106	111	116	122	127	132	137	143	148	153	158	185	211
62	104	109	115	120	126	131	136	142	147	153	158	164	191	218
63	107	113	118	124	130	135	141	146	152	158	163	169	197	225
64	110	116	122	128	134	140	145	151	157	163	169	174	204	232
65	114	120	126	132	138	144	150	156	162	168	174	180	210	240
66	118	124	130	136	142	148	155	161	167	173	179	186	216	247
67	121	127	134	140	146	153	159	166	172	178	185	191	223	255
68	125	131	138	144	151	158	164	171	177	184	190	197	230	262
69	128	135	142	149	155	162	169	176	182	189	196	203	236	270
70	132	139	146	153	160	167	174	181	188	195	202	207	243	278
71	136	143	150	157	165	172	179	186	193	200	208	215	250	286
72	140	147	154	162	169	177	184	191	199	206	213	221	258	294
73	144	151	159	166	174	182	189	197	204	212	219	227	265	302
74	148	155	163	171	179	186	194	202	210	218	225	233	272	311
75	152	160	168	176	184	192	200	208	216	224	232	240	279	319
76	156	164	172	180	189	197	205	213	221	230	238	246	287	328

Source: From www.consumer.gov.

CHARTING YOUR PROGRESS

I know you're thinking, "Not another sheet to fill in!" But, yes, unfortunately this is a must for a few very important reasons.

- Motivation is driven by success. This is not just measured by one tool, it's measured by all of the above. For example, if we just chose the scale and you gained a pound, this could totally destroy your plan. However, if you also measured yourself and did the clothes test, you may find out that you actually lost a few inches even when you gained a pound (because muscle weighs more than fat). Relying solely on the scale can leave you open to failure when you deserve success. Using a variety of tools to measure your progress can give you that all-important motivational boost from time to time—and that's something we all need to stay on track.

- Who remembers statistics? I know I don't. I barely remember what I did an hour ago, never mind last week. So make it easier on yourself by jotting down your milestones, and—even more importantly—enjoying them. Your body is shifting in the right direction, so having it on paper really does keep you going.
- Photocopy the progress chart at the end of this book, or download it from my website at www.traceymallett.com.

HOLD ONTO YOUR DREAMS

I constantly hear moms saying how their bodies will never be the same. They sigh and say, "Oh well, I'm a mom and this is what moms are supposed to look like." *What* are moms supposed to look like? In my opinion, moms should look fabulous and sexy and confident. Look in the mirror and admire yourself today. Sure, there may be a little fat here and there or bags under your eyes, but there's lots of other stuff to love about yourself. Find it and stay positive in this journey.

Keep hold of *your* goals. From my own struggles and that of my girlfriends, I know that finding time for yourself has to be a priority. Exercise can give you such a boost of energy and help keep you sane and happy amid all the craziness at home. Your body will continue to look better, your confidence will increase, and, most importantly, you'll feel like *you* again. You'll also be making a good investment in your children's future as you lead by example. Even kids as young as ten months will notice that you're enjoying exercise and learn that it should be a natural part of life, like brushing your teeth. My children work out with me all the time and they love it. They associate exercise with fun and laughter. Make it part of their lives early and they'll be more likely to continue throughout their lives.

Team Mallett Success Story

···

Melanie Wyckoff, 35, Vancouver, WA

Lost

28 pounds

4 dress sizes

17 total inches

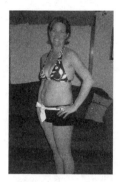
Before

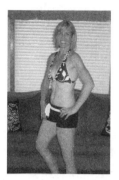
After

• • • • •

Though Melanie Wyckoff is thrilled that she lost almost 30 pounds, that's not the only benefit she reaped after having her fourth child. "Shortly after coming home from the hospital, I felt blindsided by a sudden and overwhelming sense of anxiety and constant tears," she explains. "At first, I thought it was just a heavy case of the baby blues. But then I had this feeling that I couldn't breathe or do anything but hold the baby and cry. I realized that I needed to ask for help." Despite enormous support from her wonderful husband and circle of friends, Melanie sought professional help from her doctor. "When he suggested antidepressants, I asked if I could try exercising instead. He said that that was a great idea and that studies have shown that antidepressant medications and exercise often have similar desirable effects." After just a few weeks of running and doing the workouts in the Super Fit Mama plan, Melanie felt a difference in her mood. "For me, exercise can be like a natural, healthy 'drug' that provides wonderful physical and mental results," she says. "In my case, it worked so well that I didn't need to go on medication."

Not only did the Super Fit Mama plan contribute to those good feelings, but it was easy to fit into Melanie's life no matter how hectic her schedule. "Initially, I felt overwhelmed with all of the change that needed to take place in order to look and feel fit again, but Tracey's plan makes it easy," she says. "What really helped was that the food plan is healthy and realistic, and most importantly, it's maintainable for the long haul," says Melanie. "For example, I love being able to eat unlimited veggies. I am truly never hungry." Today, Melanie is back in her pre-pregnancy clothes, and her self-proclaimed "very stretchy" stomach is taut and firm. But even more important are the mental changes. Melanie no longer feels anxious or overwhelmed. "In fact, I feel stronger and more confident than ever."

MOTIVATION FROM TEAM MALLETT

"I feel and look so much better after just three and a half weeks on the Super Fit Mama program. I've lost several inches off of my chest, hips, and legs and four pounds. My energy level is up (even on the days that I have been sleep-deprived thanks to my two-month-old), I look tighter and I feel sexy again. My husband even pinched my bottom the other day— something that hasn't happened in quite a while!"
—Ariela Chick

"In just a matter of weeks, my pooch deflated, my legs slimmed, and my second chin started decreasing."
—Jennifer Fine

CHAPTER 8

BABY
WORKOUTS
ON THE GO

YOU KNOW THOSE DAYS WHEN YOU WAKE UP FEELING TOTALLY refreshed because the baby slept soundly for eight hours the night before? Your "To Do" list is only a few items long and you have endless stretches of time to spend with your baby, exercise, and pamper yourself? Yeah, right! The baby sleeps just long enough for you to throw in a load of laundry, empty the dishwasher, and, if you're lucky, take a much-needed bathroom break. As a mom who has lived through the choppy, few-minutes-to-spare life with a baby, I've had to come up with some creative ways to sneak in exercise and lots of solutions for toning up and burning calories. The results are baby workouts on-the-go.

By using the baby as resistance—whether you're pushing a stroller up a hill or lifting him during the following strength moves—you're sure to get your heart pumping and burn baby fat fast. The good news is that with these exercises you don't have to worry about finding someone to watch your child because he or she will be right there with you. You'll be amazed how easy it is to do this and what a wonderful, fun workout partner your little one can make.

Note: Before you start the following workouts, take time to review the RPE scale in Chapter 7 so that you can safely monitor your exercise intensity. Please remember that you need to get your doctor or midwife's clearance to start any strenuous exercise.

STROLLER BURN WORKOUT

This combination walk/run workout is designed to be done with a stroller, but you can do it on your own if you actually have the opportunity to get out of the house all by yourself! The following weekly schedule starts from when you get your doctor's clearance, which is usually six weeks' postpartum.

Time: 25 minutes for one cycle; 50 minutes if you do two.

How to: Do the following sequence once; if you have time, repeat it a second time. If you do it twice, start from the 10-minute brisk walk at RPE level 5. (Of course, if your little one is getting fussy, cool down for 2 minutes and take a break. Then repeat the sequence again at a later time.)

You'll need: A comfy pair of supportive walking or running shoes.

Weeks 1–3 (after your MD or midwife gives you clearance to exercise):

5 minutes: Warm-up with a light walk at RPE 4.

10 minutes: Walk briskly at RPE 5, taking nice big strides from heel to toe. Take deep breaths as your heart rate starts to rise.

5 minutes: Light jog at RPE 6.

1 minute: Do walking lunges by stepping forward with your right leg and then bending your legs into a lunge. As you extend your legs to return to standing, lift the back leg to hip height, squeezing the glutes, and then step forward with the back leg. Repeat for 1 minute.

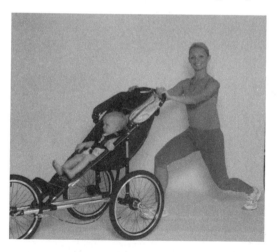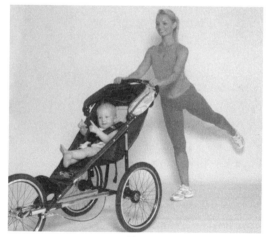

4 minutes: Cool down at RPE 4

Finish off with a kiss to your precious one to say thank you for letting you work out!

I've given you the following options to make the above workout harder as the weeks progress and you get stronger. Remember, every woman progresses differently depending on her starting level of fitness and her commitment. So don't worry if you stay with the plan outlined above for longer than three weeks. Eventually, when you feel ready, you will move on. And no matter which workout you're doing, you're still burning a lot of calories!

Weeks 4–6 (after clearance):
Do the same sequence as in weeks one through three, but decrease the brisk walk by 2 minutes and increase the light jog by 2 minutes.

Weeks 7–9 (after clearance):
Do the same sequence as in weeks 4–6, but decrease the walk by another 2 minutes and increase the jog by 2 minutes. Also, increase the jog to RPE 7.

Week 10 and beyond (after clearance):
Do the same sequence as in weeks 7–9, but increase the pace of your jog to RPE 7.5.

STROLLER TONE AND BURN WORKOUT

Time: About 28 minutes.

How to: Perform as follows with short cycles of cardio with basic toning moves.

You'll need: Your stroller and an exercise band.

5 minutes: Warm up with a moderate, easy walk at RPE 4 or a very light jog.

5 minutes: Walk briskly at RPE 5.

1 minute tone: Traveling squats with a side leg lift

Muscles targeted: Hamstrings, glutes, and quads

Reps: As many as you can do in 1 minute

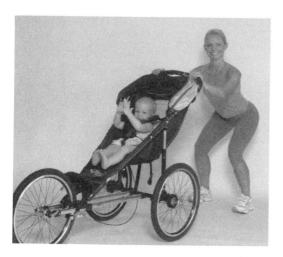 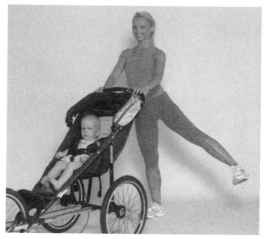

A. Start with your feet hip-width apart, knees bent in a squat position with your knees over your toes, holding onto the stroller.

B. Extend both knees and lift your left leg out to the side, hip height, leading with the heel so that your toes are pointing downward. Go back into a squat as you slightly travel forward, then lift the right leg to the side.

5 minutes: Jog at RPE 6, or if you're still not comfortable jogging, keep walking, but increase the pace by taking bigger strides.

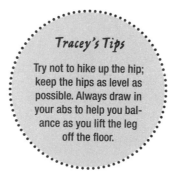

Tracey's Tips

Try not to hike up the hip; keep the hips as level as possible. Always draw in your abs to help you balance as you lift the leg off the floor.

1 minute tone: Stationary lunge with triceps extension

Muscles targeted: Triceps, glutes, hamstrings, and quads

Reps: As many as you can do for 30 seconds on each leg

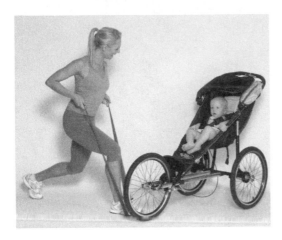 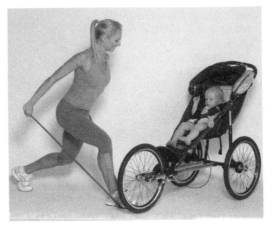

A. Stand in a lunge position with your right leg in front of you and your left leg behind you. Wrap the band under your right foot, hold onto both ends of the band, and slightly pitch the torso forward from the hips. Bend the elbows close to your sides with the elbows pointing slightly behind you.

B. Exhale and extend the elbows behind you while simultaneously bending both legs into a lunge. Next, bend the elbows and extend the legs back to start position. Repeat with your left leg forward your right leg behind you and the band wrapped around your left foot.

5 minutes: Jog at RPE 6, or if you're still not comfortable jogging, keep walking, but increase the pace by taking bigger strides.

Tracey's Tips

Keep your hand in a neutral position and your shoulders away from your ears.

1 minute tone: Super Mama's push-ups

Muscles targeted: Chest, shoulders, triceps, biceps, and abs

Reps: As many as you can do in 30 seconds

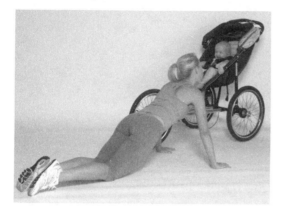
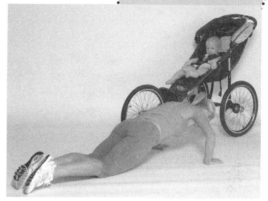

A. Situate yourself in front or to the side of the stroller with your hands shoulder-width apart on the ground and place your knees on the ground. Make sure your torso is in a straight diagonal line from your head to your knees.

B. Bend your elbows as your torso lowers to the floor, and exhale as you contract the abs, drawing the belly button toward the spine as you extend the elbows.

5 minutes: Light jog or brisk walk at RPE 5.

Cooldown: Walk slowly to gradually bring the heart rate back to normal.

QUICK POST-CARDIO STRETCH

Time: About 4 minutes.

How to: Perform each exercise once through. (If you're without baby, you can perform these exercises against a tree, wall, or chair.)

You'll need: Your stroller.

1. Glute stretch

Hold for 20–30 seconds

A. Holding onto the stroller with your arms extended, bend both knees, and lift your right leg and cross it in front of your left thigh so that your shin is resting on the thigh.

B. Sit back into your supporting heel as you open your right hip. Hold for 20–30 seconds before repeating on the other side.

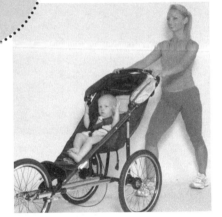

Tracey's Tips

For an extra stretch place your hand on the inside of the front thigh.

2. Calf stretch

Hold for 20–30 seconds on each leg

A. Standing tall, hold onto the stroller and extend your right leg behind you, pressing the right heel into the floor with your toes pointing straight forward.

B. Bend your front knee and slightly pitch your torso forward to further the stretch in the calves. Switch legs and repeat.

3. Hamstring stretch

Hold for 20–30 seconds on each leg

A. Hold onto the stroller with your arms extended in front of you.

B. Bend your right knee, pushing your body weight into your heel, and extend your left leg out in front of you resting on a heel as you extend your spine and hips back. Switch legs and repeat.

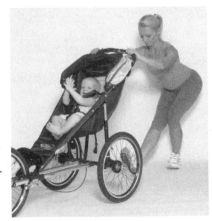

4. Back stretch

Hold for 20–30 seconds

A. Hold onto the stroller and extend both arms out in front of you.

B. Take a few steps back so that your spine is extended and you're in a straight line from your hands to your hips. Draw in the abs and hold the stretch, taking deep breaths.

Want to see how far you've pushed that stroller? Strap a pedometer on your waistband, or, better yet, keep one like the Strollometer (www.Strollometer.com) strapped to the stroller.

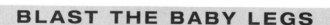

BLAST THE BABY LEGS

This workout was born—pun intended—when I found myself with my little one in a baby carrier. The extra weight from carrying her helped me to tone my legs while in transit from one chore to another. If your baby is anything like mine, it will be easy to fit this sequence in: I found that both of my kids loved movement and were at their calmest if I was slowly bobbing up and down with them. So I thought I might as well get some personal benefit and perform some leg- and butt-specific exercises. It definitely helped, so here you go—have fun on the run!

Time: About 5 minutes.

How to: Perform each exercise once through, then repeat the entire circuit a second time.

You'll need: A baby carrier (optional).

Warm-up: Walk or do knee raises in place for 3 to 5 minutes. This will warm up your lower body and get the oxygen flowing to your muscles.

1. Ballet pliés

Muscles targeted: Legs, glutes, shoulders, arms, chest, and abs

Inspiration: Dancer legs. Need I say more?

Reps: 15

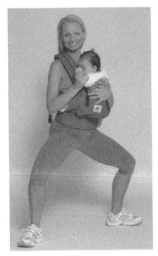

The best spot for your tot: Either in a baby carrier or in your arms. If you choose the latter, hold your baby under his armpits facing away from you, close to your chest so your elbows are bent.

A. Stand with feet a little further than shoulder-width apart, legs turned out at the hips and toes pointing out. Your knees should be over your first and second toes.

B. Inhale as you bend your knees into a plié squat. Exhale while raising your heels off the floor, then straighten your legs, lower your heels, and repeat.

Tracey's Tips

Keep your spine in a neutral position by pulling the abs in tight.

While lunging, contract the abs for balance. Counterbalance the weight of the baby by lifting your chest and drawing the shoulder blades down the back.

2. Alternating single-leg lunges

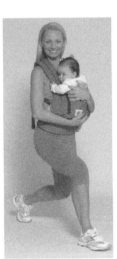

Muscles targeted: Glutes, quads, hamstrings, chest, arms, shoulders, and abs

Inspiration: To look good in those sexy yoga pants!

Reps: 10–15 on each leg

The best spot for your tot: Either in your baby carrier or in your arms. If you choose the latter, hold him against your chest as described in the first exercise in this sequence.

A. Stand with your feet together, knees relaxed, abs pulled in, and shoulders relaxed. Keep your chest lifted.

B. Take a large step forward with the right leg. Bend both knees so you're in a lunge position. Be sure to keep the right knee in line with the right ankle and the left knee pointing down to the floor. Hold the lunge for a second and then push off with the right front foot and bring your feet back together. Repeat, alternating legs.

Modification: Do this exercise while standing behind your child in a lunge position and pushing her on a swing. Return to standing after each push.

3. Standing side leg lifts with squats

Muscles targeted: Glutes, hamstrings, quads, and all the posture muscles

Inspiration: No more saddle bags!

Reps: 20 on each leg

The best spot for your tot: Either in a baby carrier or in your arms. If you choose the latter, hold him close to your torso with his face resting on your shoulder.

A. Stand with your legs together and bend the knees, with your weight resting into your heels.

B. As you extend your legs, lift the right leg out to the side just below hip height with the toe facing down to the floor, then lower the leg back into a squat position. Perform 10 reps, then repeat for another 10 reps with the toe facing up to the sky. Repeat the sequence lifting the other leg.

Tracey's Tips

Hold onto the wall, a chair, or a climbing frame at the park for support.

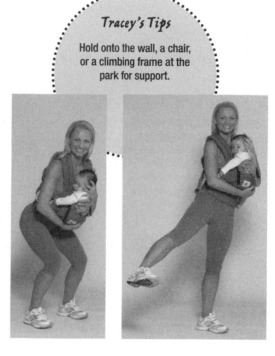

4. Lunges with leg extensions

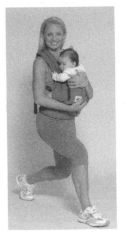
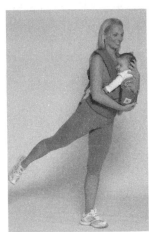

Muscles targeted: Glutes, hamstrings, and quads

Inspiration: Slimmer thighs and no more jiggle butt!

Reps: 20 on each leg (If you feel too much burn before reaching 20, take a quick break then repeat.)

The best spot for your tot: Either in a baby carrier or close to your torso with his face resting on your shoulder.

A. Stand tall, then step your right leg forward into a lunge position with both legs bent. Keep your knees over your toes and your abdominals contracted.

B. Extend the right leg by squeezing the glutes, transferring your weight onto your right leg, and lift the left leg off the floor. Then lower the leg back down and bend both legs back into a lunge, with your right leg still in front. Complete 20 reps with your right leg in front, then 20 with your left leg in front.

Modification: If this one is too difficult at first, don't lift the leg behind the body. Rest the back foot on a toe and just do the lunges.

5. Standing plié with abdominal twist

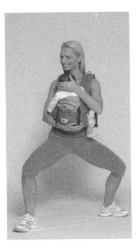
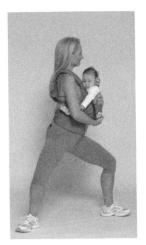

Muscles targeted: Obliques, lats, and posterior deltoids

Inspiration: No more love handles!

Reps: 10 to each side

The best spot for your tot: Either in a baby carrier or close to your torso with his face resting on your shoulder.

A. Stand tall with your feet shoulder-width apart, legs turned out at the hips and toes pointing out to the corners of the room, then bend both knees into a plié position. Place your hands in front of your baby.

B. Inhale, and then, as you twist to the right, perform two exhales. Come back to center on an inhale, then repeat to the other side.

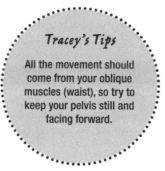

Tracey's Tips

All the movement should come from your oblique muscles (waist), so try to keep your pelvis still and facing forward.

THE DIAPER BAG WORKOUT

Many of us take our kids to the park several times per week and spend at least one to two hours pushing them on the swings or watching them crawl or toddle on the grass or slide down the slide. That's at least three hours each week when you could be burning some serious calories instead of making small talk with those moms you barely know! How? It's a cinch with what I call my Diaper Bag Workout, a name that comes from the fact that it's done with items that you can easily slip into your diaper bag somewhere between those extra clothes, diapers, and wipes. And you can do it with your child crawling around beside you, or even with him or her right on your lap. Kids love copying whatever we moms do, so while they think you're playing a game, you're actually staying fit.

Now, I know what you're going to say next because I've heard it from tons of moms I've coached. You don't want to do the Diaper Bag Workout for fear of looking like a nut in front of the other playground moms. Forget that. I guarantee that the only reason other women are looking your way is that they're curious. And remember, if they're moms, chances are that they've got a little extra flab on their abs or thighs that they want to melt, so they'll want to do it, too. Seriously, when you break the news to them that they can get fit while they let their kids get fresh air in the park, they'll think you're a genius. You can even start your own Diaper Bag Workout group!

Time: About 15 minutes.

How to: Do the following exercises in the order they appear below. Please note that where you put your baby is detailed by stages. Stage one is newborn to four months, stage two is four to nine months, and stage three is nine months and up.

You'll need: A picnic blanket and an exercise band. Bring along something to keep your little one happily entertained.

1. Seated row

Muscles targeted: Mid to upper back, biceps, and abs

Inspiration: Imagine wearing that slinky backless dress

Reps: 2–3 sets of 10–15 reps

The best spot for your tot: Stages one and two—Lying on the floor beside you or resting on your thighs. Stage three—On your lap facing you.

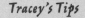

Tracey's Tips

Keep your forearms level with your elbows as you pull them back. Each repetition should be slow and controlled, working through the full range of motion.

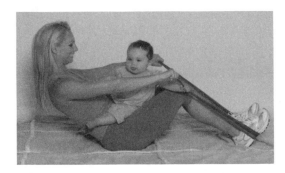 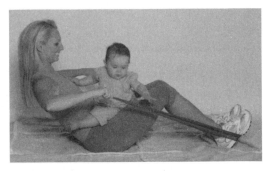

A. Sit up tall with your shoulders down and away from your ears and your chest lifted. Legs are shoulder-width apart (enough room for baby at stage one or two), stretched out in front of you with knees slightly bent. Wrap the exercise band around the balls of your feet and hold onto each end of the band. Your hands should be level with your shoulders, with your elbows slightly bent and your palms facing the floor.

B. Exhale and bring the shoulder blades down and together as you squeeze the muscles of the mid to upper back. Keep these muscles contracted as you continue to bend the elbows slightly behind the shoulder. Pause, then slowly bring the arms back in front of your body to the start position.

2. C-curl abs and bicep curls

Muscles targeted: Abs and biceps

Inspiration: Tone up your mommy-midsection flab and feel fabulous in sleeveless tops

Reps: 2–3 sets of 10–15 reps

The best spot for your tot: Stages one and two—Lying on the floor beside you or resting on your thighs. Stage three—Sitting on your pelvis.

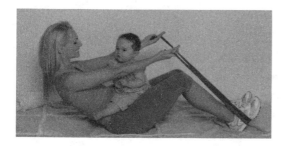 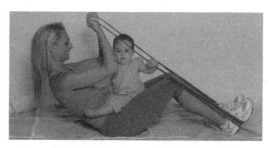

A. Start in the same position as the seated row, with the exercise band around the balls of your feet. Keep your shoulders pulled down away from your ears, your spine straight, and your arms extended, palms facing upward. Exhale, contract the abs, and slowly roll down the spine until it is in a "C" shape.

B. Keeping your torso still and your elbows in line with your shoulders, bend your elbows and bring your hands toward your ears. Pause and then straighten your arms again.

Tracey's Tips

Imagine that your upper arms are balancing a platter of food, and keep the whole body completely still with only the elbows moving. This isolates the biceps and makes the abs work hard.

3. Exercise band froggies

Muscles targeted: Quads, inner thighs, butt, hamstrings, hip rotators, and abs

Inspiration: Imagine! No more inner-thigh jiggle!

Reps: 15–20

The best spot for your tot: Stages one and two—Lying on the floor beside you or resting on your thighs. Stage three—Sitting straddled on your tummy, facing you.

Modification: Perform the exercise with your head down on the floor.

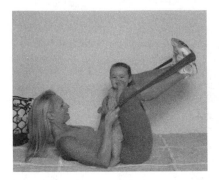 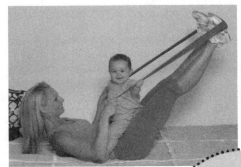

A. Lie on your back, bend your legs, and place the exercise band around the arches of your feet, elbows resting on the floor. Rotate the legs so that the heels are glued together with knees bent.

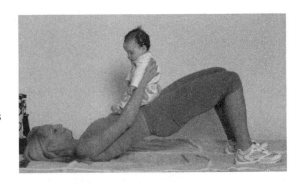

Tracey's Tips

Keep the upper body relaxed and the heels together.

B. Exhale and extend the legs out and up at a slight angle. Be sure to contract your abs and keep your back on the floor. Inhale as you bend your knees toward your ears, dropping the tailbone down toward the floor. Exhale and press your legs out against the resistance of the exercise band, getting your feet as close to the floor as possible without lifting your pelvis.

Modification: Keep head on floor.

4. Baby butt lifts

Muscles targeted: Glutes and hamstrings

Inspiration: No more cellulite!!

Reps: 20 pulses

The best spot for your tot: Stages one, two, and three—Sitting on top of your pelvis facing you. You may need to hold the baby around the waist or under the arms, depending on your child's body control.

A. Lie on your back with your knees bent, feet hip-width apart and in line with your sit bones.

B. Exhale, lift your hips off the floor, and hold a bridge position. Do a series of small pelvic tilts (little pulses contracting your glutes). I called this "the horsey" and my little one loved it!

5. Baby chair abs

Muscles targeted: Abs

Inspiration: Lose the baby bulge!

Reps: 15

The best spot for your tot: Stages one, two, and three—
Place the baby on your shins and hold him underneath the
arms.

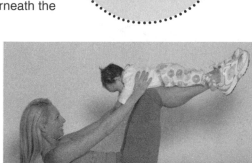

A. Lie on your back with your knees directly
above your hips, knees bent at a 90-degree
angle and shins parallel to the floor. Lift your
head, neck, and shoulders off the floor and
focus on entertaining your little one.

B. Inhale and slightly extend the legs away
from the center of your body, then exhale and
bring the knees back. Repeat for 10–15 reps
before lowering the head, neck, and
shoulders.

Modification: Keep head, neck, and shoulders on the floor.

6. Baby press-ups

Muscles targeted: Chest, triceps, biceps, and abs

Inspiration: Get rid of the tricep flab!

Reps: 2–3 sets of 10–15 reps

The best spot for your tot: Stages one, two, and three—Lying face down on top of your chest.

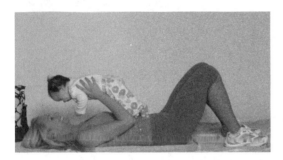 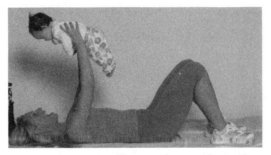

A. Lie on your back with your knees bent, hip-width apart, heels in line with your sit bones. Your elbows are bent at your sides as you hold onto your baby underneath the arms.

B. Exhale and lift the baby up above your head, extending your elbows. At the same time, draw in your belly. Focus on contracting the abs to create a stable spine. Then inhale and lower the baby toward your chest with a little kiss.

7. Super Mama push-ups

Muscles targeted: Triceps, biceps, shoulders, chest, and abdominals

Inspiration: To tone and shape your arms and give yourself a well-deserved (but scalpel-free) boob lift

Reps: 2–3 sets of 10–15 reps

The best spot for your tot: Stages one, two, and three—Lying directly underneath you, on his back.

> *Tracey's Tips*
>
> Always engage your abs, especially as you push away from the floor, so it's not just your upper body doing the work. Only go down as far as you can without moving your shoulder blades together to avoid sinking in between the shoulder blades.

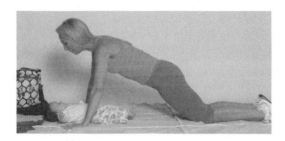 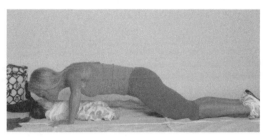

A. Place your hands directly under your shoulders, with your knees on the floor in a modified push-up position.

B. Inhale as you bend your elbows and give your child a big kiss (and watch her giggle). Then, exhale and push up.

Modification: A more advanced version is a full push-up position, balancing on your toes with your little one either seated on your back or lying directly underneath you.

8. Triceps kick back

Muscles targeted: Triceps and abdominals

Inspiration: Fabulous tank top arms!

Reps: 10–15 on each side

The best spot for your tot: Stages one, two, and three—Lying down on his back underneath you so that he can see your face.

Tracey's Tips

Keep your hand in a neutral position so as not to place any strain on your wrists.

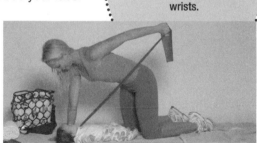

A. Situate yourself on your hands and knees with your hands directly under your shoulders and your knees directly under your hips. Place the band under your left hand on the floor and hold the opposite end with your right hand. Your elbow is bent so that your arm is resting next to your body.

B. Exhale and extend the arm, keeping the elbow close to the body, then inhale and bend the elbow. Repeat for a total of 10–15 reps before going to the other side.

9. Yoga dips

Muscles targeted: Shoulders, triceps, chest, abs, and glutes

Inspiration: Sleek-looking arms and shoulders, a strong core, and bullet-proof buns!

Reps: 5 for each leg

Tracey's Tips

Keep your shoulders away from your ears and focus on contracting the lats especially on the downward phase. Keep your abdominals tight throughout the exercise so that the spine is supported.

The best spot for your tot: Stages one, two, and three—Lying directly underneath you—the perfect spot for a quick kiss on the way down.

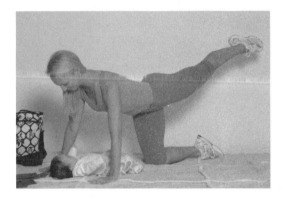

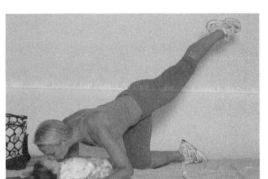

A. Start on your hands and knees, hands shoulder-width apart and knees directly under your hips, then, keeping your left knee on the floor, extend the right leg behind you at hip height.

B. Inhale and bend your elbows, keeping them close to your body so that they are pointing behind you, not to the side. The leg stays extended at hip height. Exhale, draw your abs toward the spine, and extend the elbows back to the start position.

Modification: Perform the exercise without the leg extension.

10. Side knee leg lifts

Muscles targeted: Hips and abs

Inspiration: To tone the hips and get rid of post-baby saddle bags

Reps: 15–20 on each leg

The best spot for your tot: Stages one, two, and three—Lying on the floor underneath you.

Tracey's Tips

As you move your leg keep your upper body still. Make sure your knee is going directly to the side not at a diagonal.

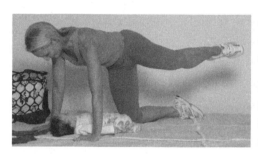

A. Start on your hands and knees with your hands shoulder-width apart directly beneath your shoulders and your hips over your knees.

B. Keeping the right knee bent, lift the right leg out to the side to no higher than hip height (try not to hike the hip up), then lower the knee and continue. Repeat on the other side.

DID YOU KNOW?

Even if you're just pushing your baby in a stroller to do your errands or around the grocery store, you're getting a workout and torching bonus calories. A recent study from the University of Wisconsin–La Crosse found that women who walked with a stroller loaded with 35 pounds burned 18 to 20 percent more calories than when they walked without one. (Though your baby may be little, his weight, your diaper bag, and all the other stuff you stash in there can easily top out at 35 pounds!) For the average woman that equals burning 375–440 calories per hour, which is equivalent to riding a bicycle at 10 mph!

11. Downward dog to plank

Muscles targeted: Chest, arms, abs, hamstrings, and calves

Inspiration: To elongate and shape your calves so they look sexy in high heels

Reps: 10–15

The best spot for your tot: Stages one, two, and three—Lying underneath you. (I can't stop my son from laughing when I do this move!)

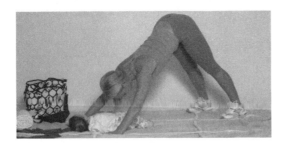

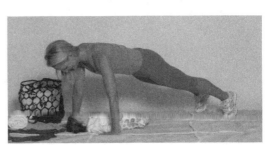

A. Stand with your feet shoulder-width apart and then reach forward and place your hands (also shoulder-width apart) on the ground. Your body should look like an inverted "V" (this is the Downward Dog pose in yoga). Press your heels down as much as possible so that you feel a stretch in your calves.

B. Without moving your hands or feet, press your hips forward toward the floor into a plank position. Pause as you say hi to your little one. Exhale, contract your abs, stay on the balls of your feet, and lift your hips to return to the "V" position.

> *Tracey's Tips*
>
> Focus on using only your abs to pull yourself up from the plank to the "V."

PUMP UP THE MUSIC

I know how hard it is to motivate yourself to work out. My number one trick for doing just that is music. Not only can you tune out, but research shows that it may inspire you to work a little bit harder. And if that doesn't rock, I don't know what does! Here are some of my favorite tunes that get me moving in the morning even after a night of interrupted sleep.

1. Madonna, "4 Minutes"
2. Seal, "If It's in My Mind, It's on My Face"
3. Christina Aguilera, "Ain't No Other Man"
4. Finger Eleven, "Paralyzer"
5. Robert Miles, "Children"
6. Duran, Duran, "Reflex"
7. Matchbox Twenty, "How Far We've Come"
8. Van Halen, "Jump"
9. Beyoncé, "Crazy in Love"
10. Wyclef Jean, "Dance Like This"

Team Mallett Success Story

Tori Takeuchi, 37, Monrovia, CA

Lost

11 pounds

2 dress sizes

11.5 total inches

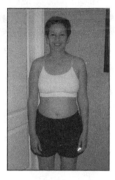
Before

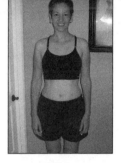
After

• • • • •

Although Tori was already at her pre-pregnancy weight when she joined Team Mallett, she really wanted to lose a few pounds and tone up. "I was used to the extra 10 pounds that I had put on since getting married, but I wasn't happy about it," she says. "And I figured that I should take advantage of my time as a stay-at-home mom to get myself in better shape."

Tori also wanted changes that went beyond how she looked. "I was feeling tired and run down and got sick easily," she says. "I really wanted to become strong and healthy so that I could be a better mom to my beautiful son." By taking part in the Super Fit Mama plan, Tori did just that.

Motivating herself to break a sweat was initially a struggle. "I've never liked to exercise, so it was tough for me to get through the workouts at first," she says. "But after just one week, I had more energy, and after two weeks, my body felt more toned and I was able to work out twice as long as I could in the beginning. Now, I actually enjoy exercising! I love that I can do the Super Fit Mama workouts in under 45 minutes and still get amazing results. And nothing beats how I feel afterward."

The food plan was a little tougher, especially when a cupcake from her favorite bakery called out to her. "But as the weeks passed, it got easier for me to say 'no' to unhealthy and fattening foods," says Tori. One reason for that is the motivation she got from seeing the numbers go down on both her scale and clothing labels. "I lost 10 pounds, which is more than I expected to lose," she says. Plus, she went from a snug size

10 to a size 8 with a little wiggle room, and she lost inches (and gained definition) in her waist, hips, arms, and legs.

"I can't believe the results I got from a program that was so short and easy to follow and that I didn't have to leave my home or spend a ton of money on," she says. "I realized that it only takes a little effort for a great reward."

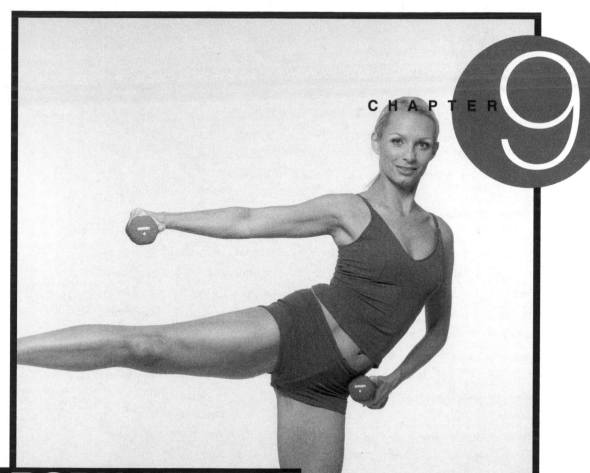

CHAPTER 9

BODY AFTER BABY PHASE II
Six Months Postpartum and Beyond

Wow, you've made it this far and you're still in the land of the living! If you have been following the plan up to this point, you've not only made it through these tough early months, but you're feeling really good. Now, don't freak out if you're not at your goal weight, because realistically you may not be. But I promise that you're getting closer. If your body still doesn't feel quite normal despite the appealing numbers you see on the scale, don't worry and don't give up. It simply takes time for you to build valuable muscle mass and time for the skin to shrink back to your new shape.

By now you're also probably wondering something that almost every woman I've trained post-pregnancy has asked me: How can I lose the extra flab on my tummy? Unfortunately, your stomach is the last section of your body to shape up. After all, think about the amazing way your skin stretched over your enormous pregnant belly—a feat that's happened more than once if you're on your second, third, or fourth child. Each time it gets stretched out, it's harder for it to bounce back to its pre-pregnancy state. It's sort of like a rubber band, which if stretched over and over again eventually starts to lose its elasticity and begins to sag. Some women naturally have more elasticity in their skin than others, thanks to genetics. Take heart that you're not alone. Even months or years postpartum, most moms have a tiny bit of the saggy skin from their pregnancy belly left over. (Yes, even celebrities; it just gets airbrushed off in pictures.) So please don't fret. The good news is that you can get your tummy in top shape with a little hard work. Take the time to understand how to use your abdominal muscles correctly with each rep you do, and you'll get the most out of every ab exercise you do. (Read "Phase I Lose Your Mommy Tummy Blast" in Chapter 7 for more detailed information on how to fully contract the abdominals.)

By now, many of you working moms are back to the grind, which will change the whole dynamics of the family and trying to fit exercise into your day. This is when the guilt starts to set in. After working all day the last thing you may want to do is take more time from your precious little one to exercise. However, you shouldn't think of exercising as taking time away from your baby—think of it as entertainment for them. When my daughter was a baby, she was quite amused by the music playing and me dancing around. When my second baby was born and Amber was two years old, she'd try to do the workouts with me. (Now that they're six and four, I have two enthusiastic workout buddies!)

Like me, Hillary from Team Mallett realized that her workouts could be entertaining for both of her kids. "Now I don't have any excuses for not doing them since my kids love watching me!" she says. For Andrea, squeezing her workouts in after her kids went to bed worked best. On a typical day, she wakes up and gets her two children ready for day care and school. She leaves the house by 8 A.M., drops the kids off, and then goes to work until 5:30 P.M., which is when she picks up the kids from day care and after-care at school. After arriving home around 6:30–7 P.M., she fixes dinner, bathes the kids, and puts them to bed, only to realize that it's already 9 P.M. Though it was late, I'm happy to report that Andrea found the time to exercise after they went to sleep, and she finally lost her last 11 pounds (read her story at the end of this chapter).

I know your children are the most important thing in the world to you, but if you don't take some time for you, then you're going to fall further and further away from who YOU really are. Your children need you to be strong and happy. I promise that if you can dedicate a little bit of time to exercise and healthy eating, you will soon look in the mirror and like what you see. Seeing how your body can bounce back after pregnancy is so inspiring. If you just take living a healthy lifestyle in stride and view it the same way you do brushing your teeth, making it part of your everyday schedule, that's exactly what it will be: part of your lifestyle and not a chore.

THE BODY AFTER BABY PHASE II WORKOUT PLAN

When you feel ready to take your workouts to the next level, it's time to start Phase II. Maybe they're starting to feel a little easier and you want an extra challenge. Remember, there is no reason why you can't mix and match the workouts. For example, maybe your arms and legs are strong enough to move on to Phase II, but your abs are still back in Phase I. No problem! In fact, the beauty of this program is that there are no rules. You're supposed to do what you can, when you can, and if for some reason you cannot do the exact workout in the program, it doesn't mean that you're not going to lose weight. It may take a little more time for you to get to your desired goal, but you WILL get there. Now, this doesn't mean that you can do just a few minutes and call it a day; it means that you should strive to do as much as you can and work out as hard as you can. It's not the time but the intensity and the consistency that will drive you to your goal. What I love about Phase II is that it's truly a workout that you can do forever!

PHASE II CARDIO STRENGTH TRAINING CIRCUIT

Time: 6 to 8 minutes per circuit.

How to: Perform each exercise once using the recommended set of weights. Repeat if you'd like to do another set. I've suggested a number of reps for each exercise, but if you are just starting out, you may start lower and work up to these targets.

You'll need: Two sets of dumbbells. (For each exercise I've indicated which set of dumbbells to use with the terms "Lighter" and "Heavier." These could be 3-lb. and 5-lb. weights, or, if you're just starting out, you might choose to use 1-lb. and 3-lb. weights instead, or 2-lb. and 4-lb. weights. If one set seems too heavy for you, go with a lighter set until you are ready to move up.)

CIRCUIT A

Warm-up: Walk around the house for a few minutes or dance with your baby. This gradually increases your core temperature and warms up the muscles.

On every exhale of each exercise, make a conscious effort to try and engage the pelvic floor.

1. Open fourth squat with overhead press

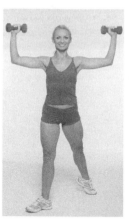 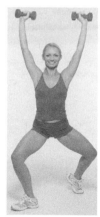

Muscles targeted: Glutes, quads, hamstrings, calves, shoulders, and abs

Inspiration: Toned legs and shoulder definition!

Reps: 12 on each leg

Weights: Lighter

A. Start with your legs turned out at the hips and your toes pointing out to the corners of the room. Your right leg is positioned in front of the left leg about 3 feet at a slight diagonal (imagine a diagonal line from your left heel to your right heel), and your left leg is resting on the ball of the foot with the heel elevated. Bend your elbows so they're level with your shoulders.

Tracey's Tips

Focus on keeping your knees over your toes and drawing your shoulder blades down to the hips. Keep the tailbone tucked under so that you don't overarch the lower spine.

B. Bend your knees into a squat with your knees over your first and second toes while extending your arms overhead, then extend your legs and bend your elbows back to the start position. Do 10 reps before repeating with the other leg in front.

Modification: Perform the exercise without elevating your heel for a more stable base.

2. Side kick triceps extension

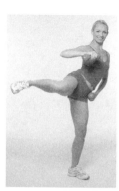

Muscles targeted: Glutes, quads, hamstrings, and triceps

Inspiration: Say goodbye to saddle bags and flabby arms!

Reps: 10 on each leg

Weights: Lighter

A. Stand on your left leg, which is slightly bent, and the right knee extended to the side so that your right knee is level with your right hip. Bend your right elbow so that it is level with your shoulders; and your palm is facing downward.

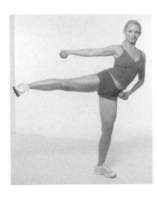

B. Extend the right leg out to the side to hip height so that you're leading with the heel and the toe is pointing down to the floor. At the same time, extend your right arm out to the side level with the shoulder. Next, bend the knee and elbow back to start position. Complete 10 reps then repeat to other side.

Modification: If balance is an issue, hold onto the wall or a chair.

Note: Place weights on the floor.

Tracey's Tips

Always turn your toes down to the floor so that your focus is on the glutes, not the quads.

Always land toes first, then lower the heel all the way to the floor, bending the knees slightly to minimize the impact on your joints.

Cardio:

Jump out and in for 60 seconds.

Muscles targeted: Quads, hamstrings, glutes, and calves

Inspiration: Blast lower body fat!

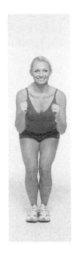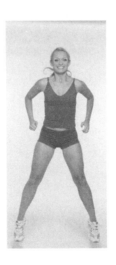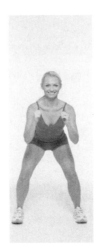

A. Start with the feet together, knees bent in a squat and arms bent beside your hips.

B. Jump out to a wide squat with your weight in your heels, then back to start position. Use your arms to propel yourself into the air.

Modification: If you have any back or knee problems, keep one foot on the floor at all times rather than jumping.

3. Lunge rotation to row

Muscles targeted: Mid to upper back, obliques, quads, hamstrings, and glutes

Inspiration: To get rid of back fat, tone the waist, and lift the butt!

Reps: 10 on each leg

Weights: Heavier

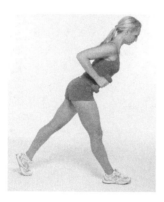 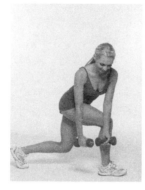

A. Start in a lunge position with your right leg in front of you and the left leg behind, resting on the ball of the foot, knees bent. Rotate your upper body toward the right (front) leg with both arms reaching toward the floor.

B. Exhale and draw the shoulder blades together as you bend your elbows behind you in a row and simultaneously move into an upright position.

Modification: Perform the move without the rotation and simply do the row.

4. Present and side ski

Muscles targeted: Biceps, shoulders, quads, hamstrings, and glutes

Inspiration: Beautiful arms and shoulders and gorgeous thighs!

Reps: 15–20

Weights: Lighter

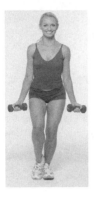 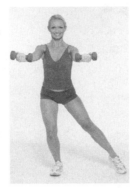

A. Start with your legs together, right leg bent resting on the ball of the foot, arms by your sides with your palms facing forward.

B. Spring to the right, bring the left foot to the right foot, and rest the left foot on a toe as you lift your arms to shoulder height, palms facing forward, then lower the arms to the start position. Alternate the legs for 15–20 reps.

Modification: Just step to the side without a spring.

Note: Place weights on the floor.

Repeat cardio:

Jump out and in for 60 seconds.

CIRCUIT B

1. Side lunge fly with fly and tricep extension

Muscles targeted: Quads, hamstrings, glutes, triceps, and mid to upper back

Inspiration: Toned back, flawless arms and legs!

Reps: 10 on each side

Weights: Lighter

Tracey's Tips

Keep the torso slightly pitched forward from the hips and draw the shoulder blades down to avoid stress in your neck and shoulders.

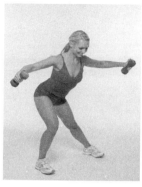
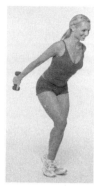

A. Start with your feet shoulder-width apart, toes pointing forward, and your arms slightly rounded with the palms facing toward each other. Step out to the right side and bend the right knee, extending the left leg into a side lunge. Make sure your knee is over your toes; your torso is slightly pitched forward from the hips. At the same time, extend your arms to the sides, leading with the elbows, to activate the mid to upper back.

B. Draw your left leg to meet your right leg and rest foot on toe, with your elbows bent behind your torso. Next, do a tricep extension and alternate for a total of 20 reps, then repeat on the other side.

2. Single leg squat row

Muscles targeted: Mid to upper back, glutes, hamstrings, and quads

Inspiration: Improve your balance and tone the butt!

Reps: 10 on each leg

Weights: Heavier

Tracey's Tips

Focus on drawing in your abdominals so you are balancing from a strong core.

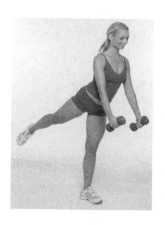
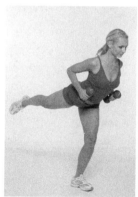

A. Start with your right leg about two feet off the floor, extended behind you. Your arms are extended forward palms facing inward.

B. Exhale and draw the shoulder blades together as you bend your elbows behind you in a row. At the same time, bend your supporting leg, making sure the knee is tracking over the toes. Do 10 reps, then repeat on the other side.

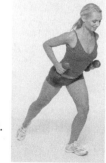

Modification: Either perform this exercise with your leg resting on your toes or eliminate the squat.

Note: Place weights on the floor.

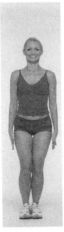
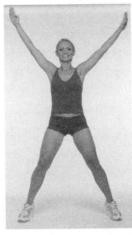

Cardio:

Good Old Jumping Jacks for 60 seconds.

Inspiration: Burn lots of calories!

A. Start with your legs together and your arms by your sides.

B. Jump as you open your legs a little further than hip-width apart and lift the arms into a high "V" position. Then jump again and bring the legs back together as you lower your arms back down beside your body.

Modification. If you have knee, back, or any joint issues, do right and left side taps, reaching the opposite arm across your body, instead of jumping jacks.

3. Plank to side plank

Muscles targeted:
Total body

Inspiration:
Madonna's yoga body!

Reps: 6 on each side

Weights: None

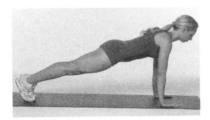
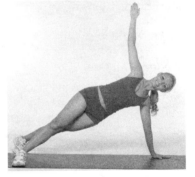

A. Start with your arms shoulder-width apart, with your hands on the floor directly under your shoulders and your legs extended, so that you are in a plank position with your abs contracted for support.

B. Twist your torso to the left as you open the left arm up to the ceiling so that your hips and torso are facing left. Lower your hand and twist your torso back to the plank position, then repeat to the other side. Alternate sides for a total of 6 reps on each side.

Modification: Bend the leg that is on the same side as the supporting hand and lower the knee to the floor for more support.

Tracey's Tips

Try not to sink in between the shoulder blades, and keep drawing the shoulder blades down toward the pelvis in order to keep any tension out of the head, neck, and shoulders.

4. Lunge with big arm circles

Muscles targeted: Quads, hamstrings, glutes, shoulders, and biceps

Inspiration: Total body tone up!

Reps: 10 on each leg

Weights: Lighter

Tracey's Tips

Do not lift the arms any higher than the shoulders, and keep drawing the shoulder blades down toward the hips.

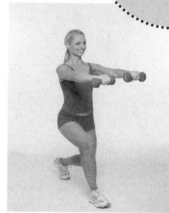
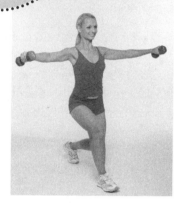

A. Start with your right leg in front of you and your left leg behind you in a lunge position. Place your arms at your sides with your palms facing toward the back of the room.

B. Bend both knees and lift your arms straight forward to shoulder height, then open them to the sides, palms facing downward. As you extend the legs, lower the arms back to their start positions. Repeat for 10 reps, then reverse the arm circles with the other leg in front.

Note: Place weights on the floor.

Repeat cardio:

Repeat Good Old Jumping Jacks for 60 seconds.

CIRCUIT C

1. Side lift attitude with shoulder raise

Muscles targeted: Shoulders, biceps, quads, hamstrings, glutes, and calves

Inspiration: Dancer's legs and arms!

Reps: 12 on each leg

Weights: Lighter

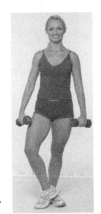 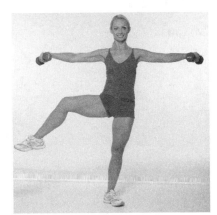

A. Start with your legs turned out at the hips so that your toes are pointing out to the corners of the room and lift your heel off the floor resting on the ball of the foot. Round your arms in front of you and rest your hands on your thighs.

B. Lift the right leg out to the side, leading with the knee so that your right thigh is at hip height. As you do this, raise your arms out to the side at shoulder height, leading with the elbows. Lower the leg and arms back to start position and repeat for a total of 8 reps on each side.

Modification: Instead of lifting the leg, simply keep the foot still.

Tracey's Tips

Focus on drawing in the abdominals and contracting the glutes on the supporting leg as you lift the opposite leg for stability. Try not to hike up your hip as you lift the leg.

2. Row with external rotation

Muscles targeted: Mid to upper back and rotator cuff

Inspiration: Strong shoulders to avoid shoulder injuries from toting baby!

Reps: 10

Weights: Lighter

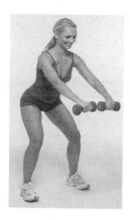
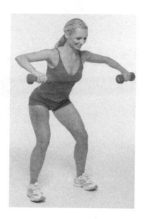
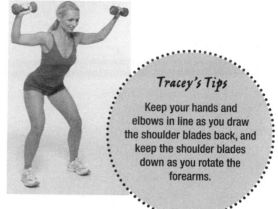

Tracey's Tips

Keep your hands and elbows in line as you draw the shoulder blades back, and keep the shoulder blades down as you rotate the forearms.

A. Start with your feet shoulder-width apart and your knees bent in a squat with your torso slightly pitched forward from the waist. Your arms are in front of your chest with your palms facing downward.

B. Inhale as you bend your elbows and squeeze your shoulder blades together. Then exhale and rotate the forearms up so that your palms are facing forward and your elbows are directly under your wrists. Return to the start position and repeat.

Modification: Perform the move with one arm at a time, with the opposite hand resting on the thigh.

Note: Place weights on the floor.

Cardio:

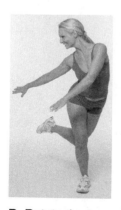
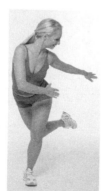

Ski Rotation for 60 seconds.

Muscles targeted: Glutes, hamstrings, quads, and obliques

Inspiration: Blast lower body fat and shrink the waist!

A. Start with the legs shoulder-width apart, knees slightly bent, then step out to the right side and bend the left knee behind the body.

B. Rotate the torso and arms toward the right side. Then push off the right leg and spring out to the left side, bringing the right leg behind the left and twisting the torso toward the left side. Alternate sides for 30 seconds.

3. Push-ups with leg extension

Muscles targeted: Chest, shoulders, abs, and glutes

Inspiration: Upper body and mommy-tummy make-over!

Reps: 8 on each side

Weights: None

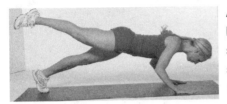

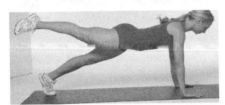

A. Start with your hands on the floor, shoulder-width apart, arms straight, and your legs extended behind you in a push-up position. Lift the right leg off the floor to hip height.

B. Inhale and bend your elbows as you move your torso toward the floor, then exhale as you draw your abs toward the spine and straighten the elbows. Repeat, holding the leg up at hip height, for 8 reps, then lower the leg. Repeat with the left leg lifted.

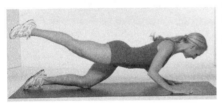

Modification: Look at the Phase I version and perform on a chair for elevation to make the exercise easier.

4. Curtsey side lift with overhead press

Muscles targeted: Shoulder, quads, glutes, hamstrings, and calves

Inspiration: Beautiful toned butt and shoulders!

Reps: 12 on each side

Weights: Lighter

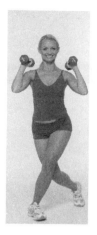 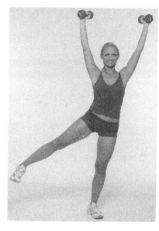

A. Start with the right leg diagonally behind you in a curtsey lunge with your hips facing forward as you bend both legs. Your elbows are bent so that your hands are by your shoulders with your palms facing in.

B. Extend both knees and lift the right leg off the floor and out to the side. At the same time, extend your arms over your head with the palms still facing toward each other. Then bend your right knee as you return to the curtsey lunge. Do 10 reps before switching to the other side.

Modification: If balance is an issue, then just take the working leg to a point and not lift it off the floor.

Note: Place weights on the floor.

Cardio:

Repeat Ski Rotation for 60 seconds.

Tracey's Tips

Contract the supporting leg, especially the glutes, to enable you to balance. Also, try not to hike your hip up as you lift your leg off the floor.

PHASE II LOSE YOUR MOMMY TUMMY BLAST

Time: 6 to 8 minutes.

How to: Perform one set of each exercise.

You'll need: A rolled-up towel or exercise band and a pillow.

1. Pelvic bridges with figure eights

Reps: 5 each direction

Inspiration: Tight abs and toned hamstrings!

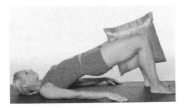 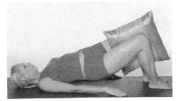

Tracey's Tips

Focus on squeezing the pillow and drawing up your pelvic floor throughout the figure eight.

A. Place a pillow between your knees and lie on your back with your knees bent and your feet hip-width apart. Your heels are in line with your sit bones, and your hands are by your sides.

B. Exhale as you draw in your abs and do a pelvic tilt, rolling up through the spine until you're in a bridge position.

C. Tilt the pelvis toward the right side and move up and around, making a sideways figure eight. (The middle of the eight is the starting bridge position.) After performing five in each direction, slowly roll down through the spine, breathing space in between each vertebra until you're lying on your back in a neutral spine position.

2. Abs towel pulse in chair position

Reps: 10 exhalations with pulses

Inspiration: To finally understand how to achieve flat abs with breathing (what a concept)!

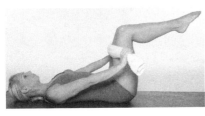

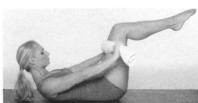

Modification: See Phase I version.

A. Lie on your back with your knees directly above your hips, knees bent at a 90-degree angle and shins parallel to the floor. Squeeze your inner thighs together and place the rolled-up towel in front of the thighs, holding it taut with your hands at the sides of your thighs.

Tracey's Tips

Keep your knees directly over your hips, fighting the resistance of the towel pushing in the opposite direction. Your focus should always be on pulling in the abdominal wall, not pushing out. Try adding a "Quick Flick" Kegel with every exhale (see Chapter 2).

B. Exhale, drawing in the abdominals and lifting your head, neck, and shoulders off the floor. Hold this position as you perform 10–12 tiny up-and-down pulses, then roll back down.

3. Towel-resisted scissors

Reps: 10 on each leg

Inspiration: Flexible legs and toned midsection!

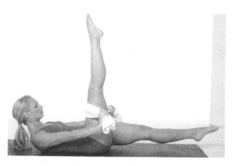

A. Lie on your back with your knees directly above your hips, knees bent at a 90-degree angle and shins parallel to the floor. Place the rolled-up towel in front of your thighs with your hands holding onto each end to create resistance. Contract the abs as you pull your knees toward your chest and push the towel in the opposite direction. Lift your head, neck, and shoulders off the floor.

B. Exhale as you lower the right leg down to the floor so that it's hovering a few inches off the ground, while the left leg is against the towel, pushing toward the chest. Switch legs on an inhale and repeat for a total of 10 reps on each leg.

Modification: Slightly bend the knees, or keep your head, neck, and shoulders on the floor.

Tracey's Tips

Keep your upper body still rather than moving it toward each leg. Focus on resisting the towel and pulling in the abdominals.

Imagine that your hip and lowest rib on each side are pulling together as you twist the pelvis.

4. Lower abs curl with twist

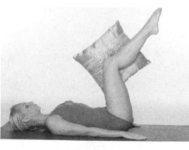

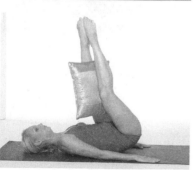

Reps: 8 on each side

Inspiration: No more lower belly pooch!

A. Place a pillow between your inner thighs and lie on your back with your hands by your sides. Your legs are slightly bent and extended up to the ceiling.

B. Exhale and draw your abdominals toward the spine, lifting the hips off the floor into a pelvic tilt. Continue to exhale as you twist toward the right side, and then come back to center as you lower the hips on an inhale. Repeat, twisting toward the opposite side.

Modification: Perform without the twist. Follow the version of this exercise in Phase I (Chapter 7).

5. V-sit twist with canoe

Reps: 10 on each side

Inspiration: Tiny Tummy!

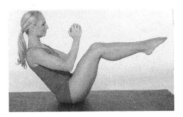 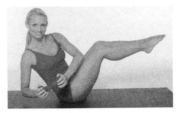 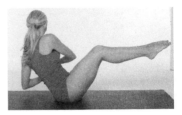

A. Start by sitting tall with your legs bent at a 45-degree angle in front of you and your shins parallel to the ceiling. Extend your spine so that you're balancing on your tailbone and your body forms a "V" position. Extend your arms and clasp your hands together, or hold a light dumbbell in front of your chest at shoulder height.

B. Keeping the hips and legs still, exhale and twist the torso to the right as your arms circle down to the floor and up back to center. Your body twists through center on an inhale. Exhale as you repeat the movement on the other side. Your hands are making a sideways figure eight.

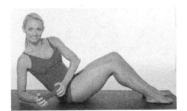 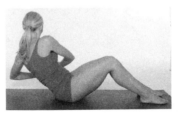

Modification: Perform the exercise with your feet on the floor and your legs bent.

Tracey's Tips

Keep your focus on your hands to increase your rotation and work the obliques (waist) more. It's important to breathe throughout the exercise.

Keep your hips stacked and facing forward throughout the exercise.

6. Side plank lifts with side leg lift

Reps: 10 on each side

Inspiration: Strong legs and rock-hard abs!

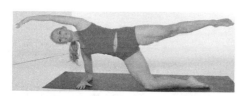

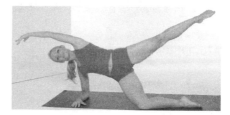

A. Start by sitting on your right hip with your right leg slightly bent and your left leg extended straight out. The inside of your left foot is resting on the floor in front of the right foot. Balance your upper body on your right forearm with your elbow bent and directly underneath your shoulder as you draw your shoulder blade down toward your hips, releasing stress in the upper body.

B. Exhale and lift your hips off the floor as you reach your left arm up and over into a side stretch. At the same time, lift the left leg to just a little higher than hip height, pause, and then gently lower your hips back down. Repeat 10 times before going to the other side.

Modification: Keep both knees bent.

7. Run in forearm plank with twist

Reps: 10 on each leg and 10 twists

Inspiration: Tight fitting tank top!

Tracey's Tips

Imagine that your pubic bone is moving toward the belly button as you scoop out your belly into a pelvic tilt. This will intensify the abdominal contraction. Try to keep your shoulders over your elbows at all times.

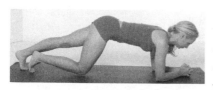

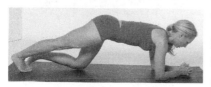

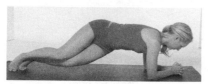

A. Balance on your forearms with your shoulders over your elbows, your legs extended behind you, and your toes turned under. You should be in a straight line from the crown of your head to your heels.

B. Bend the right knee and then the left, slowly picking up the pace into a "run." Keep your shoulders over your elbows. Contract the abdominals the whole time and exhale every time you bend your knee.

C. With the legs together, twist the torso and the knees toward the right and then quickly twist to the other side. Alternate sides for a total of 10 reps.

Modification: Hold the plank position for 30 seconds without moving the torso.

PHASE II MAMA BUTT BLAST

Time: 6 to 8 minutes.

How to: Perform one set of each exercise.

You'll need: Light to medium-intensity exercise band. (The exercises can be done without the exercise band if you prefer.)

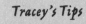

Tracey's Tips

Keep the band taut at all times to work the lower body muscles the whole time. Ouch!

1. Step side grand pliés

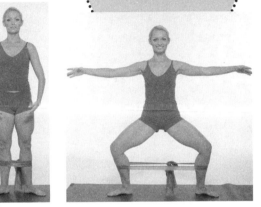

Muscles targeted: Glutes, quads, and hamstrings

Inspiration: Got rid of thigh wobble fast!

Reps: 12 on each side

A. Wrap your band tightly around your calves and tie it in front. Turn your legs out at the hips so that your feet are in a small "V" position (ballet first position). Extend your arms out to your sides, slightly rounded at shoulder height.

B. Step your right foot out to the side a little further than shoulder-width apart into a deep plié (or as far as you feel comfortable), making sure your knees are over the toes as you lift your arms. Transfer your weight to the right leg and return to a small "V" position with your feet, extending the legs and lowering the arms back to the start position. Do 12 reps, then repeat to the other side.

Modification: If balance is an issue, hold onto a chair for support or plié without the transfer back to a "V" position.

2. Elevated donkey side kick

Muscles targeted: Glutes, hamstrings, and quads

Inspiration: To make cellulite a thing of the past!

Reps: 10 extensions and 10 pulses

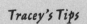

Tracey's Tips

Keep the hips stable by drawing in your abs, and try not to sink in between your shoulder blades. Keep the arms straight and strong and the hips square.

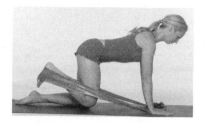 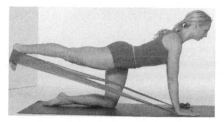

A. Start on all fours with your hands directly under the shoulders and your knees directly under your hips. Wrap the exercise band around your right foot and hold the ends of the band in your hands. Lift one knee about 8 inches off the floor, flexing your foot, and extend the leg toward the back wall.

B. Push your heel out behind you as you extend the leg to hip height. Repeat for 10–15 reps, then hold the leg at hip height and pulse up and down for 10–15 reps. Lower the leg and repeat the sequence to the other side.

Modifications: Perform the version in Phase 1 without the pulses or without the exercise band.

3. Side kicks with circles

Muscles targeted: Glutes, quads, and hamstrings

Inspiration: No more maternity pants!

Reps: 10 on each leg with 8 circles forward and 8 backward

Tracey's Tips

Make sure your knee is never higher than your hip. Keep the knee and shin parallel to the floor as you bend toward chest with your hips stacked and facing forward. Lift up out of the floor and try not to sink in the shoulders.

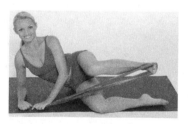 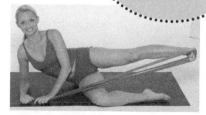

A. Lie on your right hip with your right elbow bent, balancing on the forearm. Wrap the band around the left foot, holding the ends of the band in front of your chest on the floor, and bend your knees slightly with the left leg at hip height.

B. Extend the left leg, leading with the heel. Be sure to keep your knee in line with the hip. Repeat for 10 reps, then perform small, controlled circles forward and backward before going to the other side.

Modification: Perform without the band for less intensity.

4. Glute blasters!

Muscles targeted: Glutes

Inspiration: A perky dancer's butt!

Reps: 20 with 20 tiny pulses

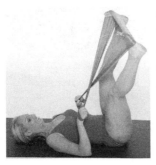

A. Lie on your back with your legs extended up to the ceiling and your toes slightly turned in toward each other. Wrap the band around both feet, cross it in front of your legs, and hold onto the ends in front of your chest. Your elbows are resting on the floor on either side of your torso.

B. Leading with the heels, slightly open the legs a little further than hip-width apart and then return to the start position. Repeat for 20 reps, then perform tiny pulses.

5. Swimming with rotation

Muscles targeted: Upper and lower spine, glutes, hamstrings, and obliques

Inspiration: Beautiful toned back, hamstrings, and butt.

Reps: 20 on each side

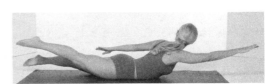

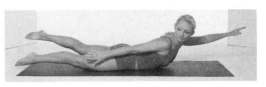

A. Lie on your front with your upper body extended off the floor and your right arm extended over your head level with your right ear. Your left arm is beside your body level with your hip. Lift the legs as you press the pubic bone to the floor.

B. Reach your left hand down toward your feet as you side bend the upper body toward the left side. Start to flutter kick the legs as fast as you can for 10–20 reps, then switch the arms, side bend toward the right side, and repeat.

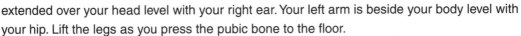
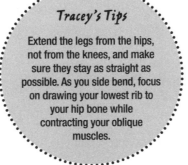

6. Starfish

Muscles targeted: Glutes, hamstrings, upper and lower spine

Inspiration: Toned back and booty!

Reps: 20

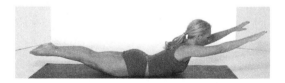 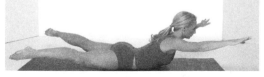

A. Lie on your front with your upper and lower body extended and lifted off the floor. Turn the legs out at the hips so that your heels are together in a small "V" position and extend your arms over your head in line with your ears.

B. Exhale, open the legs to hip-width apart, and open the arms into a "V" position. Inhale and return the arms and legs back to the start position. Repeat, staying high in the spine extension.

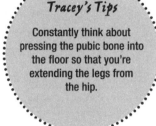

Tracey's Tips

Constantly think about pressing the pubic bone into the floor so that you're extending the legs from the hip.

Modification: Bend your elbows and place your hands by the sides of the rib cage and do the legs only.

SUPER FIT MAMA FLEXIBILITY SEGMENT

Perform the Flexibility Segment from Phase I (see Chapter 7).

CIRCUIT A

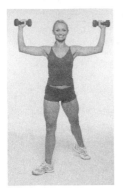
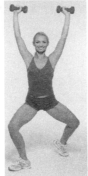

1. OPEN FOURTH SQUAT WITH OVERHEAD PRESS

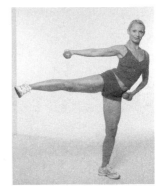

2. SIDE KICK TRICEPS EXTENSION

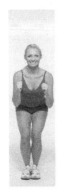
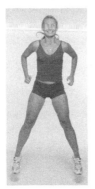
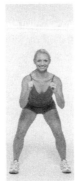

CARDIO: JUMP OUT AND IN FOR 60 SECONDS

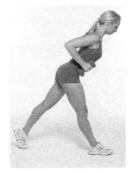
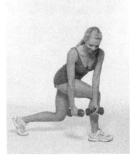

3. LUNGE ROTATION TO ROW

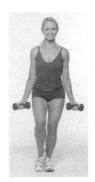
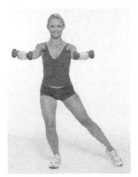

4. PRESENT AND SIDE SKI

CARDIO: REPEAT JUMP OUT AND IN FOR 60 SECONDS

CIRCUIT B

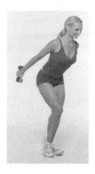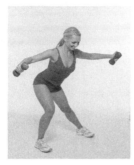

1. SIDE LUNGE FLY WITH FLY AND TRICEP EXTENSION

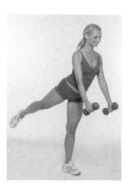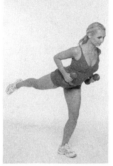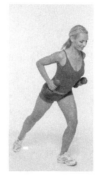

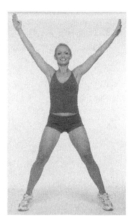

2. SINGLE LEG SQUAT ROW **MODIFICATION** **CARDIO: JUMPING JACKS FOR 60 SECONDS**

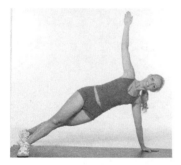

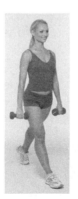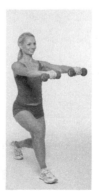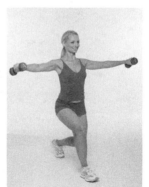

4. LUNGE WITH BIG ARM CIRCLES

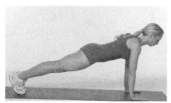

3. PLANK TO SIDE PLANK **CARDIO: REPEAT JUMPING JACKS FOR 60 SECONDS**

CIRCUIT C

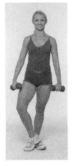

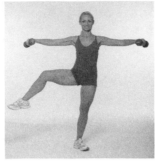

1. SIDE LIFT ATTITUDE WITH SHOULDER RAISE

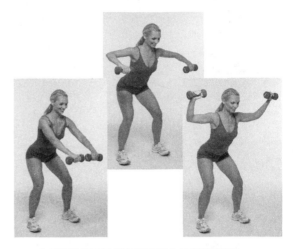

2. ROW WITH EXTERNAL ROTATION

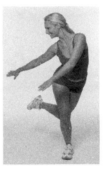

CARDIO: SKI ROTATION FOR 60 SECONDS

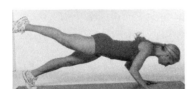

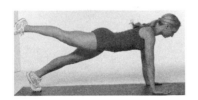

3. PUSH-UPS WITH LEG EXTENSION

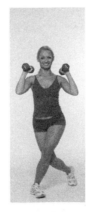

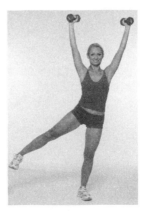

CARDIO: REPEAT SKI ROTATION FOR 60 SECONDS

4. CURTSEY SIDE LIFT WITH OVERHEAD PRESS

PHASE II LOSE YOUR MOMMY TUMMY BLAST

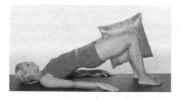 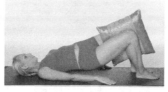

1. PELVIC BRIDGES WITH FIGURE EIGHTS

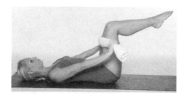 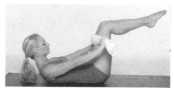

2. ABS TOWEL PULSE IN CHAIR POSITION

3. TOWEL-RESISTED SCISSORS

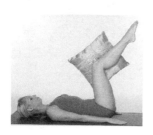 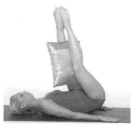

4. LOWER ABS CURL WITH TWIST

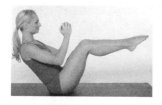 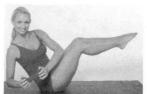 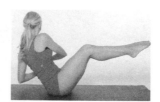

5. V-SIT TWIST WITH CANOE

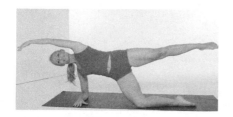 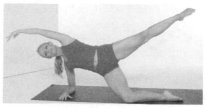

6. SIDE PLANK LIFTS WITH SIDE LEG LIFT

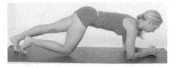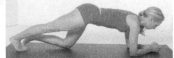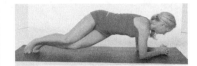

7. RUN IN FOREARM PLANK WITH TWIST

PHASE II MAMA BUTT BLAST

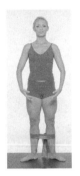

1. STEP SIDE GRAND PLIÉS

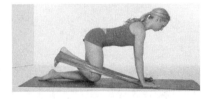
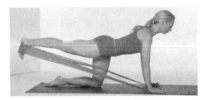

2. ELEVATED DONKEY SIDE KICK

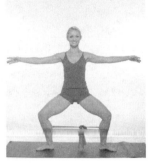

3. SIDE KICKS WITH CIRCLES

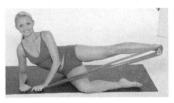

4. GLUTE BLASTERS!

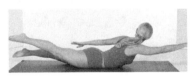
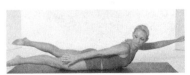

5. SWIMMING WITH ROTATION

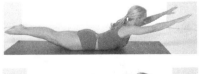
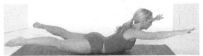

6. STARFISH

CARDIO TIME

I know there's a lot of talk in the fitness world about the "fat burning zone" and that getting there means long workouts at a low intensity. It's correct that during those workouts the primary fuel source is fat; however, they do nothing to boost your metabolism. We're programmed to believe that when it comes to losing weight, more cardio is the preferable choice. Yes, you will burn a lot of calories that way, but often at the cost of utilizing the precious muscle mass that you need to keep your metabolism running at high gear. Who has the time to do an hour of cardio a day when you can work for a shorter amount of time at a higher intensity, preserving valuable muscle mass with less impact on your joints? At this rate you will be working harder for a longer amount of time without the same results. The Super Fit Mama plan recommends 20–30 minutes of cardio workouts three times a week, just enough to exercise your heart and burn some calories.

Initially, in Phase I, starting to do cardio again may be challenging for you, and at that point just moving the body at a good pace to a RPE level of 5 or 6 is advised as you build up your strength. However, now that you're in Phase II, you should be able to add a few aerobic intervals (short bursts of high-intensity cardio) into whatever type of cardio you choose to do, whether it's a walk, run, jog, or swim. You can start off with shorter intervals—like 1 minute—and then pick up your pace to go at a high effort for 2 minutes at a time, and return back to a comfortable pace for 5 minutes. As you get stronger, those 2-minute intervals will become

BENEFITS OF INTERVAL TRAINING

1. It saves time. You don't need to do more than 20–30 minutes to get an effective and efficient workout compared to 1–1.5 hours of exercising at one steady pace.

2. It's better for your joints. Because the high-intensity intervals are done for a shorter amount of time, your joints aren't exposed to as much wear and tear. I recommend performing cardio interval workouts three or four times a week for best results.

3. Interval training increases your metabolism. It does so because it is believed to give you a post-exercise calorie burn that lasts up to twenty-four hours after your workout (something that does not happen if you exercise at one steady pace).

4. Interval training can be adapted to weight training, exercise machines, and medicine ball workouts. It keep the workouts fresh, fun, and challenging. Also, because you're only pushing for short amounts of time, you feel a sense of accomplishment as it's doable.

5. Studies suggest that interval training stimulates a greater release of growth hormone, which helps to build lean muscle mass.

longer and your recovery intervals shorter. In my opinion, you don't need to do any more than 20–30 minutes of cardio if you're performing intervals, which is essentially what the Super Fit Mama workouts are.

If you continue doing the same workout for months on end without changing it, your body gets bored and won't change as quickly. At this point, since your goal is to lose the baby fat, you need to stress your muscular and cardiovascular system beyond what it's normally accustomed to (going to a point where you're breathless for a short period of time) to improve it. Doing this on a regular basis will enable your body to in turn burn more calories during and after the workout.

Success Story

Andrea Frye, 36, Alhambra, CA

Lost

14 pounds
2 dress sizes
11 total inches

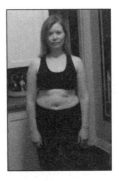
Before

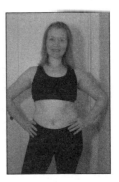
After

After the birth of her second child, Andrea felt horrible. "My clothes didn't fit and I didn't have the energy to play with my new baby and five-year-old daughter," she says. "Even worse, I lacked confidence and, as a result, all I wanted to do was stay home and hide rather than go anywhere." Luckily, she heard about the Super Fit Mama plan, which was exactly "the push I needed to get off the couch and start working out." In fact, not only did Tracey get Andrea off that couch, she made her eager to work out.

"Though at times it's hard to figure out when I'm going to fit in a workout, the plan is so fun that it makes me want to do just a little more each time," she says. Though one hard part of slimming down for Andrea is maintaining a healthy diet and avoiding impulse eating decisions, being on a structured program helped. "I work full time and have two kids, so Tracey's recipes make it much easier for me to eat healthily, and the food plan means that I don't really have to think about what to eat," she says. "I still struggle with my cravings, but now instead of *automatically* reaching for chocolate, I stop and ask myself, 'Do I really need that?' Most of the time, the answer is no." Still, Andrea has learned that it's okay if the answer is occasionally yes. "This program isn't about starving or depriving yourself," she says. "It's about making healthier choices." The good news is that these better choices are not just helping Andrea. "They infuse into my family's life as well. After all, when I'm eating better, my oldest daughter and husband do the same," she says.

All her hard work has certainly paid off. "Typically, no one says anything about the way I look, but since Tracey's program I've had a lot of positive comments from family and friends," she says. "Someone even said that I'm losing too much weight—I've never heard that before!" Though she's thrilled that she can fit back into her pre-baby clothes and "feel ab muscles instead of a flabby middle," it's what Andrea's *gained* that makes her hard work well worth it. "I feel so much better about myself and have regained my confidence and energy," she says. "I enjoy looking in the mirror and seeing the happier person looking back at me."

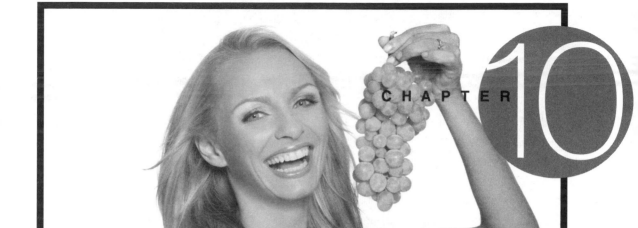

CHAPTER 10

EATING FOR ONE AGAIN
Postnatal Nutrition

KNOW YOU'RE ANXIOUS TO GET OUT OF THOSE MATERNITY CLOTHES and feel slim again, but let me just say that the first month postpartum is no time to diet or even restrict what you eat. Your body has gone through a lot over the past nine months (after all, it just created and pushed out another human being!), so the last thing it needs is to be cut off from important nutrients. Instead, it needs time to heal and have the energy to care for a newborn (which you've probably realized is no easy feat!). On top of that, experts say that limiting food portions for the first three weeks after the birth can interfere with breastfeeding and milk production. That said, sticking to mostly healthy foods will keep you from feeling too fatigued and help you regain your energy and heal.

Once the first month has passed, you can start changing your diet. If you were on the Super Fit Mama program while you were pregnant, then you're familiar with the basics of healthy eating and just have to make a few changes now that your little one has arrived. If you're just starting the program, no worries. It's simple to understand and doesn't require a major diet overhaul. After all, I'm a mom, too, and I know that a life of nibbling salads with dressing on the side is both boring and inadequate; it's not going to give you even a fraction of the energy you need to keep up with your growing baby.

SUPER FIT MAMA'S EATING PLAN MAIN POINTS

1. A balance of healthy fats, fibrous and complex carbohydrates, and lean protein along with an abundance of fruits and veggies is your winning ticket for weight loss and management.
2. Eat every three hours to keep your metabolism burning. This means having six to seven small meals a day, such as breakfast, mid-morning snack, lunch, mid-afternoon snack, dinner, and an optional evening snack. Try not to let yourself go hungry. This will keep your blood sugar level and prevent you from overeating at your next meal.
3. Do not skip breakfast. Breakfast is the most important meal of the day to get the metabolism going. As the name implies, you eat this meal in order to break the ten to twelve-hour fast you've had from eating since the night before.
4. Drink between eight and twelve glasses of water daily. The upper amount is essential for milk production, especially since you're exercising. Water is essential to keep your milk production at its premium.
5. Always have pre-prepared snacks on hand. Take a few hours on the weekend to portion out your snacks so that you have a variety to choose from when you're in a rush, or when your sugar level dips and you need a quick pick-me-up. If you start delving into the actual snack boxes, two crackers end up being six and an ounce of cheese ends up being five ounces. Believe me, I've been there: Don't leave any stone unturned for temptation.
6. Be sure to get those important omega-3 essential fatty acids found in fish, flaxseeds, omega-3 fortified eggs, and nuts. To avoid getting too much mercury, limit your intake of shark, tile fish, king mackerel, farmed salmon, and swordfish to once a month. And only eat nuts if neither you nor your partner has a family history of nut allergies; if your baby has inherited a risk for a nut allergy, early exposure through breast milk could increase that risk further.

If you're breastfeeding, in some ways you are still eating for two, so the need for good nutrition is just as important. If you're drastically cutting calories, you will not be able to get enough of all the required nutrients your body needs at this time and your milk supply will suffer. Also, it's hard to get the required daily amount of calcium in low-calorie food choices. And if you're not getting enough calcium, your bones will be stripped of this important ingredient for milk production, leaving you at risk for osteoporosis later on in life.

On the other end of the spectrum, some women use breastfeeding as an excuse not to slim down. But research from the University of Iowa shows that modest weight loss doesn't affect your milk production. If you're breastfeeding, you need to up your caloric intake by about 300–500 calories a day, just like during pregnancy. You should also make sure these are nutrient-rich food choices, not nutritionally empty ones.

Whether or not you are nursing, you need to wait at least four to six weeks post-delivery before beginning a weight-loss program that restricts calories and includes strenuous physical activity. You need all the energy you can get to recover from giving birth. If you're nursing you should lose no more than 1 pound a week after the first month (unlike 2 pounds a week for non-nursing moms). Yes, I know this is a hard thing to comprehend when you're looking in the mirror with your belly on vacation, but every woman's body is unique and the weight will come off at different times. Fat cells seem to be very resilient after childbirth; they're hanging around in case we should have a famine or you get pregnant again. You can't change nature—the fat cells are there to protect your milk supply. Drastically cutting calories will only make them hold on even more, so eat small meals at least every two to three hours and, most importantly, exercise when you have your MD's go-ahead, following the postpartum plans outlined in previous chapters.

Despite the fact that you're tired of feeling big and frustrated about how your body looks, don't view food as the enemy. Instead, remind yourself that food is your source of the vitamins and minerals that will keep your body strong and energetic and protect you from illness. The right kind of nutritious foods will actually help you lose weight, not gain more.

Remember, too, that it took you nine months to gain the weight, so how can you expect to lose it all in six weeks? That said, if you follow this plan, I promise that you will see the former you emerging in just four to five months' postpartum in a safe, effective, and healthy way. Team

Mallett saw results in a matter of weeks. Not only did these moms have more energy, but they became much more optimistic and more motivated to get back into shape. Attitude is everything, so repeat after me, "I can do this and I will be a Super Fit Mama!" The more you say positive affirmations, the more you will believe you can reach your goal.

THE SUPER FIT MAMA FOOD PLAN

This is a healthy eating plan, not a *diet*. To most, the word "diet" means starvation, and you know by now that this is not our goal. The Super Fit Mama food plan is a healthy way of eating that you can use forever, not just to shed your baby weight. With this plan you can indulge, but also learn how to control portions.

When you're breastfeeding and your body is trying to heal from the marathon of pregnancy, labor, and delivery, you need to eat nutritious foods. Not only will junk food keep those pregnancy pounds on long past your baby's first birthday, but it will leave you feeling sluggish (and new moms don't need any more fatigue) and bad about yourself. Low self-esteem is not helpful when you're juggling life with a newborn. At times, you may think that something sugary will give you a boost because you feel tired, but it will really just give you an energy crash. Instead, when a craving hits, take a deep breath and step away from the junk food. Better yet, don't keep any junk foods in the house. Remember that you have just brought a new life into the world, and in order to look and feel your best you need to eat right. The nutrients found in fruits, veggies, and whole grains can impact your mood in a positive way and have been known to help regulate hormones. And if there's ever a time you need help with raging hormones, it's in this postpartum period.

I've tried my best to make this eating plan so simple that even a sleep-deprived, hormonal new mom can follow it. I've done so by listing the foods and exactly how much you should allow yourself. The key here is all about portion control. By eating smaller portions more often throughout your day, you'll naturally control how many calories you eat—no math required!

I've also made sure that many of the foods in my plan work double duty to slim you down while giving you the nutrients you need to ward off disease, enhance your energy, and help you look your best. The first week or two, you will likely need to measure your food or weigh it, but soon enough you'll learn what a correct portion size is and be able to

I'm a mother of twins and breastfeeding. How many more calories do I need to consume?

Add an extra 500–600 calories per day for each child you're nursing, depending one whether you're exclusively breastfeeding or supplementing with formula.

Should I be eating fewer calories when my baby starts eating solids?

It's hard to determine what your caloric needs are going to be as one baby's demands for milk will differ from another's. I suggest you go by your hunger level in between meals. Also, if you still need to lose weight and you're having difficulties losing up to a pound a week, then this will be your indicator to decrease you calorie intake. If you're doing the 2,300-calorie plan, then go down to the 2,200-calorie plan and monitor your weight loss, and so on.

Is it safe to eat sugar substitutes?

This debate has been going on for a long time. After an incredible amount of research, the Center for Science in the Public Interest has decided that Splenda (sucralose) is a safe alternative. All the other substitutes are probably best avoided, especially if you are breastfeeding. Saccharin has been linked to many cancers in rats, and the National Cancer Institute found some evidence of increased risk of bladder cancer in heavy saccharin users. (Heavy is six or more sugar substitute packets or 16 ounces or more of diet soda daily.) Stevia is an herbal sweetener from the stevia plant that has not yet been approved as an additive by the Food and Drug Administration (FDA). Although it is natural, there is not enough evidence yet to suggest whether it's safe to use through pregnancy or when nursing. It is not advised to use any herbal supplements during pregnancy.

In my opinion plain old sugar—in moderation—is not bad for you. The U.S. Department of Agriculture suggests a limit of ten teaspoons of added sugars per day for people who eat a 2,000-calorie diet. This is equivalent to about one 12-ounce soft-drink. American diets consist of way too much sugar, but you have the power to control the amount of sugar you eat.

I love coffee. Is it safe to drink it when I'm nursing?

Caffeine does pass into your milk supply and can cause your baby to be irritable and extremely alert all hours of the night (not something a new mom wants!). But here's a solution: Only drink one or two cups of coffee a day, and keep your caffeine intake to less than 300 milligrams. Remember, it's not just coffee that contains caffeine; tea, soda, and chocolate all do as well.

Try switching to decaffeinated coffee and tea as an alternative, and save chocolate as a small treat. I do not recommend drinking herbal teas during pregnancy, however, as their effects on the developing fetus have not yet been determined.

What is all this hype about high-fructose corn syrup? How do I avoid it in my diet?

You're right to be concerned about HFCS, which is usually found in baked packaged goods, cakes, candy, fruit drinks, cookies, and sodas, but it doesn't stop there. You can find it in foods that you would not expect, such as salad dressing, sauces, peanut butter, and some canned goods. Many experts believe that the increase in its use has contributed to our obesity problem because HFCS can be addictive, catering to your sweet tooth and leaving you wanting more and more. The result is consuming more calories. Manufacturers use HFCS because it's a lot cheaper than cane sugar to produce—and it's also even sweeter as it's made from cornstarch. Animal studies have found a link between increased consumption of HFCS and diabetes, and HFCS also seems to raise cholesterol levels. It's imperative to limit your consumption of HFCS, not only for your health and weight maintenance but for your children. Make it a point to check food labels.

eyeball it on your own. What's interesting about these first few weeks is that you'll be amazed to see what a true portion is compared to how much you were eating before. After all, portion sizes in this country have gotten huge over the past twenty years, so we think heaping plates of food are normal. Then when we see a correct portion we think it's a meal made for a mouse. Trust me, it's not. You'll actually realize that you're full and satisfied on a lot less food than you may be used to.

Here are some tips to keep in mind as you follow the Super Fit Mama plan:

1. If you're breastfeeding, you will serve your little one between 400 and 700 calories in breast milk on a daily basis. Milk production alone requires in the region of 800 calories daily. So even if you did no physical activity your body would need more calories just to make the milk. Experts suggest that you increase your calorie intake by 500 calories from your pre pregnancy

HIDDEN CONTAMINANTS

Every day we're exposed to contaminants, and unfortunately it can get into our breast milk. Breast milk is partly made from the fat supplies sitting on your hips, abs, and thighs, and though you are longing to slim those body parts down quickly, losing too much weight too quickly has been associated with the release of environmental contaminants stored in body fat into the milk. This is why I must remind you again to lose no more than 4–5 pounds a month for safe weight loss after the first month of delivery. It's also imperative that you do your best to avoid environmental exposure as much as possible. The first step is your diet, as it plays an important role in protecting your baby from the chemicals that can accumulate in breast milk and potentially be harmful to your baby. Keeping the level of contaminants in your breast milk as low as possible involves following a few commonsense rules:

- Avoid alcoholic beverages.
- Eat a balanced diet low in animal fats and avoid high-fat dairy products.
- Trim all visible fat off meats because dioxin (a chemical contaminant) accumulates in fat.
- Eat lots of fruit and veggies as they contain little dioxin.
- Eat organically grown food, when available, or locally grown produce. Buying at the local farmers' market is a great way to get your produce and support local farmers at the same time.
- Avoid fish that may have high mercury or PCB levels, as mentioned in Chapter 5.
- Scrub your produce with water or a veggie cleaner.
- Peel waxed fruit and vegetables such as apples, pears, cucumbers, and peppers.
- Always eat a varied diet so that you're limiting your exposure to any one food.

When all is said and done, scientists and medical professionals all agree that a diet that is low in animal fats and high in organic fruits, veggies, and grains is not only better for you and your baby, but better for the environment.

daily amount. You want to be on the low end of that range if you're supplementing with formula and/or solid food, and the higher end if you're exclusively breastfeeding.

2. Avoid drastically cutting calories for the first four to six weeks after giving birth. At this point, your most important goal should be to settle in to your new life with your baby and take time to heal.

3. Never go below 1,800 calories per day if you're breastfeeding. You would not be able to get all the necessary nutrients into your body with a smaller amount. For formula feeding mamas, a minimum of 1,600 calories is recommended.

4. The easiest way to determine how many calories you need is to listen to your body, eat healthy when you're hungry, and drink when you're thirsty. A safe range for breastfeeding mamas greatly depends on your weight and your activity level. Monitor your weight loss and milk supply. If you're losing more than a pound a week and your milk is slowing down, increase your calories. However, if you're not losing, then reduce your calories a bit. Eventually you will find a balance.

5. If you are a vegetarian, consider taking a vitamin supplement containing vitamin B12, as a B12 deficiency can be detrimental to your baby's development. If you don't eat any dairy products, make sure you get enough calcium from other sources. Your doctor or midwife will probably advise you to continue taking your prenatal vitamin as long as you are lactating, especially if you are a vegetarian or vegan. The American Dietetic Association recommends that vegan women eat sources of alpha-linolenic acid such as flaxseeds, soybean oil, canola oil, and tofu to increase the amount of alpha-linolenic acid in their breast milk.

6. Water plays a huge role in your milk production. You will need to drink at least eight to twelve glasses of H_2O spread out throughout the day. Have a big glass of water while breastfeeding or right afterward. Amazingly, those of us who breastfeed exclusively can produce between 750 and 800 milliliters of milk a day, so staying hydrated is key! I always kept a bottle of water on the side table next to my rocking chair where I would

breastfeed. Another tip: Place a glass of water with ice cubes next to the chair where you'll do your middle-of-the-night feeding. By the time this comes around, you'll have a nice refreshing glass of water to sip.

7. Keep taking your prenatal vitamin. Nursing moms need 1,000 milligrams of calcium and at least 200 IU of vitamin D every day from food and supplements to keep their bones healthy.

8. Eat carbs. Low-carb diets actually hinder milk supply and can have negative effects on the quality of your milk.

9. You may no longer be pregnant, but getting all the important nutrients and food groups into your diet is crucial for your breast milk and your health. And many nutrients also help speed up weight loss. (Now I've got your attention!) See Chapter 5 for detailed info on all these nutrients and why you need them.

HOW THE PLAN WORKS

Table 10.1 shows you how to allocate your food portions depending on your daily total calorie plan. This will ensure you're eating a balanced diet by giving you the correct amounts from all the food groups.

Breastfeeding mamas need 500 calories more than their pre-pregnancy daily calorie count. Find your daily calorie intake with Table 10.1 and use this as a guide for your meal plan. You should never go below 1,800 calories. Experts agree that 2,000 calories and up is a much safer calorie range. This will allow you to get all the essential nutrients that you need to help protect your body and produce milk for your baby. And chances are, your doctor will tell you to keep taking your prenatal vitamins or a good multivitamin.

Non-breastfeeding mamas can follow the lower amounts on the chart. I recommend that you do not go below 1,600 calories a day, as your body needs energy and valuable nutrients to repair and replenish itself. You can gradually cut the calories later if you are not losing pounds, but give yourself at least a few weeks to recover from labor and delivery.

TABLE 10.1: DAILY SERVINGS BY FOOD GROUP BASED ON CALORIE INTAKE FOR POSTPARTUM MOTHERS

CALORIES*	PROTEIN	DAIRY	GRAINS	VEGGIES	FRUIT	FATS
1,600	7 P	3 D	6 G	Unlimited	4	3
1,700	7	3	7	Unlimited	4	4
1,800	7	3	8	Unlimited	4	4
1,900	7	3	9	Unlimited	4	4
2,000	7	3	9	Unlimited	4	5
2,100	7	3	10	Unlimited	4	5
2,200	7	3	11	Unlimited	4	6
2,300	7	3	12	Unlimited	4	6
2,400	8	4	12	Unlimited	4	7
2,500	8	4	13	Unlimited	4	7

*Caution: Breastfeeding mamas should NEVER go below 1,800 calories.

SUPER FIT MAMA FOOD PORTIONS

PROTEIN

High-protein foods can range from 35 to 100 calories per serving.

Note: Some protein entries include "+ *one fat.*" These foods have a high enough fat content that you should count them as one serving of protein and one serving of fat on your food planner. See also separate lists below for beans and lentils as well as for nuts, which are also high in protein.

Poultry
1 oz. chicken or turkey, light meat, without skin
1 oz. chicken or turkey, dark meat or with skin, + *one fat*

Fish
1 oz. catfish
1 oz. haddock
1 oz. mahi mahi
1 oz. salmon
1 oz. sea bass
1 oz. sole
1 oz. canned salmon, packed in water, not oil
1 oz. canned tuna, packed in water, not oil

Shellfish

1 oz. clams

1 oz. crab

1 oz. imitation shellfish

1 oz. lobster

1 oz. scallops

1 oz. shrimp

Beef

1 oz. beef (USDA select or choice grades
of lean meat with visible fat trimmed.
Grass-fed beef is the ultimate choice.)

1 oz. beef with 15–20 percent fat, + *1 fat*

1 natural organic beef, turkey, or pork hot
dogs, + *1 fat* (Try to avoid regular hot
dogs whenever possible because they
often contain nitrates, which are thought
to cause cancer, as well as MSG and
preservatives.)

Pork

1 oz. lean pork

1 slice Canadian bacon

3 slices bacon, + *one fat* (Cut off all fat,
not only for the calorie content but for
possible contaminants that may be
stored in the fat.)

Lamb

1 oz. lamb (roast, chop, or leg)

Soy

½ cup tofu

¼ cup tempeh

1 soy hot dog

Eggs

1 whole egg

2 egg whites

¼ cup egg substitute

Cheese

1 oz. reduced-fat cheese (American, cheddar, feta, goat, Monterey jack, Swiss,
part-skim mozzarella)

1 oz. regular cheese, + *1 fat*

½ cup low-fat cottage cheese

2 tablespoons grated Parmesan cheese

¼ cup (2 oz.) fat-free or low-fat ricotta

1 oz. soy cheese

Other

1 tablespoon natural peanut butter, almond
butter, or other nut butter, + *one fat*

GOING ORGANIC

Organic food definitely tastes better and is believed to be a better choice for you as well as for the environment. Although organic foods can be more costly than their nonorganic counterparts, prices have been coming down as the demand has risen, particularly in the category of organic frozen fruits and veggies. Don't shy away from frozen foods; the nutritional content is comparable to that of fresh produce and they're great to have at hand for a quick stir fry. Always look for the USDA organic seal on foods, a sign that a product is at least 95 percent organic, or look for "made with organic ingredients," which means that the product has at least 75 percent organic ingredients.

DAIRY

Dairy foods range from 100 to 160 calories per serving.

Note: Some dairy entries include + *one fat*. These foods have a high enough fat content that you should count them as one serving of dairy and one serving of fat on your food planner. (Cheeses are listed in the Protein section above.)

Milk
1 cup fat-free milk
1 cup 2% fat milk, + *one fat*
1 cup fat-free or low-fat soy milk
1 cup fat-free or low-fat yogurt
Preferred brands: YoMommy low-fat organic yogurt, made by Stonyfield Farm, has added folic acid, vitamin D, and DHA.

VEGGIES

Half a cup of cooked or 1 cup of raw veggies in the non-starchy category equals 25 calories. For starchy veggies, see list of grains.

Artichoke
Artichoke hearts (packed in water)
Arugula
Asparagus
Bean sprouts
Beets
Broccoli
Brussels sprouts
Cabbage
Carrots
Cauliflower
Celery
Chilies
Cucumber
Eggplant
Green beans
Green onions
Leeks
Mushrooms
Onions
Peppers
Radishes
Salad greens
Spinach
Tomato
Turnips
Watercress
Zucchini

FRUITS

Fresh or frozen fruits are about 60 calories a serving.

1 small apple (4 oz.)
½ cup unsweetened applesauce
4 apricots
1 small banana
¾ cup blackberries
¾ cup blueberries
1 cup cubed cantaloupe
12 (3 oz.) fresh cherries
3 dates
½ large grapefruit (11 oz.)
1 cup (3 oz.) grapes
1 cup (10 oz.) cubed honeydew
1 kiwi
¾ cup fresh mandarin orange sections
½ small mango
1 small nectarine
1 small orange
½ or 1 cup cubed papaya
1 medium peach (4 oz.)
½ large fresh pear (4 oz.)
¾ cup cubed fresh pineapple

2 small plums (5 oz.)
3 prunes
2 tablespoons raisins
1 cup raspberries
1¼ cup strawberries
2 small tangerines
1¼ cup cubed watermelon
2 tablespoons dried fruits

Unsweetened Fruit Juice
Note: Choose natural juices with no added sugar. Whole fruit is a better choice than fruit juice because it contains more fiber. Try to consume fruit first!
½ cup apple juice
⅓ cup cranberry juice
½ cup grapefruit juice
½ cup orange juice
½ cup pineapple juice
⅓ cup pomegranate juice

GRAINS AND STARCHY VEGGIES

Generally, one serving of grains equals around 80–100 calories, give or take a few. You might be wondering why I've placed some vegetables under this category; this is purely because of the calorie content.

Note: Some grain entries include + *one fat*. These foods have a high enough fat content that you should count them as one serving of grain and one serving of fat on your food planner.

Whole-Grain Breads

1 slice of whole-grain bread (Look for the whole-grain seal to make sure you're actually eating whole grain, and look for bread with at least 3 grams of fiber per slice.)

½ English muffin (100 percent whole grain)

½ 6-inch-round whole-wheat pita bread

½ small hamburger or hot dog bun

1 6-inch-round whole-wheat tortilla

¼ slice naan bread

½ whole-wheat bagel

1 small, plain, whole-wheat dinner roll

1 cup whole-wheat baked croutons

4-inch whole-grain waffle

1 2½-inch biscuit, + *one fat*

1 small plain muffin, + *one fat*

1 2-inch cube cornbread, + *one fat*

2 4-inch diameter pancakes, + *one fat*

Pasta and Grains

½ cup cooked whole-grain pasta

⅓ cup cooked brown rice

½ cup cooked quinoa (6 tablespoons dry)

½ cup cooked couscous

3 tablespoons wheat germ

⅓ cup hummus, + *one fat*

3 cups plain air-popped popcorn

½ cup chow mein noodles, + *one fat*

Preferred brands: Barilla Plus, Ronzoni Healthy Harvest

Whole-Wheat Crackers (preferred choice)

4 ak-mak brand whole-wheat crackers

4 Wasa Fiber Rye crackers

Cereals

⅓ cup dry oatmeal (steel-cut is the most nutritious)

½ cup cooked barley

⅓ cup bran cereal (All Bran, Bran Buds, Fiber One)

½ cup bran cereal, flaked

½ cup cooked bulgur

¼ cup low-fat granola (less than 10 grams of fat per serving)

½ cup cooked kashi

½ cup cooked millet

½ cup or 1 biscuit shredded wheat

1½ bricks Weetabix

⅓ cup other unsweetened cereal

Preferred brands: Nature's Path

Note: Check the nutritional panel on foods. A serving size of 15 grams equals one bread serving.

A study from the University of North Carolina found that breastfeeding moms who were overweight didn't affect their milk production even when they slashed 500 calories from their diets and lost weight.
Eat slowly and chew your food. This will allow the brain to tell you when it's full so you don't ingest too many calories.

Other Crackers and Snack Foods

8 animal crackers

8 small pretzels

3 2½-inch square graham crackers

4 slices melba toast

5–6 saltine crackers

20 oyster crackers

15–20 fat-free or baked chips

2 large ricc cakes or 6 mini rice cakes (look for the types made from brown rice)

11 soy chips

4–6 whole-wheat crackers (no fat added)

4–6 whole-wheat crackers with fat added, such as Triscuits, + *1 fat*

Beans and Lentils

The following foods are a great source of protein (for example, 1 cup of beans has 12 grams of protein, a perfect choice for vegetarians), but I placed them in the grain section because of their calorie content.

⅓ cup lentils

½ cup baked beans

½ cup cooked beans, such as black beans, chickpeas (garbanzos), kidney beans, lima beans, pinto beans, or split peas

Starchy Veggies

1 small baked or boiled potato

1 cup cooked winter squash (butternut or acorn) and/or summer squash

½ cup yam or sweet potato

½ cup green peas

½ cup corn (or ½ ear of corn)

½ cup plantain

½ cup jicama

1 cup vegetable broth

1½ oz. French fries, + *one fat*

Energy Bars

½ of an approximately 200-calorie bar

½ Lara bar (www.larabar.com)

½ BellyBar (www.nutrabella.com)

½ Fiber One chewy bar

½ Luna bar

1 Pria bar

Other Starchy Foods

1 tablespoon sugar, honey, maple syrup, corn syrup, jam, or jelly

½ cup marinara pasta sauce, + *one fat*

¼ cup fat-free salad dressing

3 cups popped popcorn (no fat added)

FATS

Healthy fats have around 45 calories per serving. To help reduce calories, always try to use low-fat options when available.

Oils

Note: The following list has the preferred options.

1 teaspoon of the following oils:

Canola

Corn

Macadamia

Extra virgin olive

Sesame

Seeds

1 tablespoon of the following:

Flaxseed, ground

Pumpkin

Sesame

Sunflower

⅛ of an avocado

Nuts

Note: Pregnant women with a history of allergic reactions can minimize the risk to their children by avoiding certain known allergens, especially tree nuts (cashews, almonds, pecans, and walnuts) and peanuts. Breast-feeding mothers should also avoid foods that contain these allergens, as they can be transmitted to babies via breast milk.

1 tablespoon or ¼ cup of the following:

Almonds

Cashews

Peanuts

Pecans

Walnuts

8 olives

½ tablespoon of natural peanut butter, almond butter, or cashew butter

2 teaspoons tahini

Other Fats

1 tablespoon olive or canola-based salad dressing

2 teaspoons reduced-fat salad dressing

1 tablespoon reduced-fat margarine

1 teaspoon regular mayonnaise

2 teaspoons light mayonnaise

1 teaspoon butter

2 teaspoons light margarine

1½ tablespoons reduced-fat cream cheese

3 tablespoons reduced-fat sour cream

FREE FOOD

Note: As long as you don't eat excessive amounts of the following condiments, there's no need to record them.

Broth, low-sodium
Mustard
Salsa
Soy sauce
Taco sauce

Tomato ketchup
Vinegar
Wine, used in cooking sauce
Worcester sauce

THE FOOD LOG

The food log makes the Super Fit Mama plan especially easy. I know many women who ignored the food log for weeks until they couldn't understand why they were not losing the last five pounds. Initially after your baby is born, just exercising more and eating a well-balanced diet will help you lose those excess pounds quickly. However, as you get closer to your goal, this advantage will start to slow down, and it's at this time that knowing exactly what goes into your mouth and being accountable for it will make a huge difference. I know that I often pick from my kids' plates, but that can add up to a few hundred calories a day. To combat this I make extra veggies and eat those instead of the pizza crust.

If you really want to slim down, you need to start off on the right track. Simply put, if you don't write down exactly what and when you're eating, you're relying on remembering every morsel of food—something that "Mommy brain" does not allow for. I really felt like I lost a million brain cells after having my first child, then it tripled after the second. You have to write everything down—even when you're on the go (a small purse-sized notebook is perfect for this). It may seem like a royal pain at first, but trust me, this will save you lots of calories and help curb the mindless eating that happens when you've got kids.

Keeping the food log is easy. Below I provide a sample that you can use as a guideline. It shows you how many foods from each group to eat, depending on how many calories you need per day. For every portion you eat, place the corresponding letter in the food box. For example, 1 medium-sized apple is 1 fruit, so you mark off one F. If you eat a slice of whole-wheat bread, this is 1 grain, so you will mark off one G. You will be referring often to the list of portions and sizes provided above in this chapter.

Photocopy the blank Food Log from the back of the book (or print it out from my website at www.traceymallett.com), and you're ready to go. Now don't dodge it, I want you to be successful! Also, it's important to follow these guidelines as closely as possible and not skimp on any of the nutrients, since all of them are important for staying full, slimming down, and building strong, lean muscles.

Example—TEAM MALLETT SUPER FIT MAMA MEAL LOG 1900 CALORIES

	Protein	Dairy	Grains	Fruits	Fats	Veggies (nonstarches)	Water
Breakfast	P P P P P	D D	G G G	F F	F F	V V V	W W
Snack	P P P	D D	G G	F F	F	V V V	W
Lunch	P P P P P	D D	G G G	F	F F	V V V	W W
Snack	P P P	D D	G G	F F	F	V V V	W
Dinner	P P P P P	D D	G G G		F F	V V V	W W
Evening snack (optional)	P P P	D D	G G	F F	F F	V V V	W
Day's Maximum	7	3	9	4	4	Unlimited	8
DAY'S TOTAL	Ate 7 portions of protein	Had 3 Diary foods	Had 9 lots of grains	Ate 4 pieces of fruit	Had my 4 FATS allowance	Had loads 'n' loads of veggies	Drank at least 8 glasses of water

Daily Notes: Feeling good today my pants are starting to feel looser.

*See resource section for a copy of the food log for you to photocopy or go www.traceymallett.com and download it.

I also recommend that you write down some other valuable information—the kinds of things that will help you identify stressful situations, increase your awareness of foods that make you feel more satisfied, and let you know what times of day you need to be prepared with healthy treats because you tend to get hungry then.

Each log should include the following.

1. The times you ate.
2. The times you were the hungriest.

WHY ARE WHOLE GRAINS SO IMPORTANT?

I can't stress enough how important it is to switch to whole grains because they contain filling fiber and healthy nutrients. White bread is stripped of the bran and germ portions of the plant, losing valuable fiber, phytochemicals, and vitamin content. Fiber is your winning ticket for weight loss. Also, research shows that whole grains can reduce your risk of disease: stroke by 30–60 percent, type 2 diabetes by 21–30 percent, and heart disease by 25–28 percent. A recent study even suggested that women who ate large amounts of fiber reduced their risk of breast cancer by an amazing 50 percent. The problem is that most of us don't get close to the RDA of three servings daily (16 grams is one serving).

I know it can be difficult figuring out what is whole grain and what is not—you can't just go by the color and think that just because it's brown, it's whole grain. You have to be diligent and read the labels. I'm a big fan of getting a good portion of my whole grains in at breakfast time. I love Natural Path Organic Bran, which is available in most grocery stores, mixed with granola and pumpkin seeds and topped with berries. This makes for a perfect highly nutritious breakfast in seconds. You can substitute other brands of bran flakes. When you go to the supermarket, look for these popular whole grains:

- Amaranth
- Barley
- Buckwheat
- Bulgur
- Corn, including whole cornmeal and popcorn
- Millet
- Oats, including oatmeal
- Quinoa
- Rice, brown rice, wild rice, and other specialty rices (as long as it is not white!)
- Rye
- Wheat

Typically, you can count something as a serving of whole grains if it contains 16 grams of whole-grain ingredients. Here are some examples of one serving of easy-to-find whole-grain foods:

- 4 Triscuit crackers
- ⅔ cup Cheerios
- one slice whole-grain bread
- ½ whole-grain English muffin
- ⅓ cup cooked whole-wheat pasta
- ⅓ cup cooked brown rice, bulgur, barley, or other cooked grain

An organization called the Whole Grains Council issues "Whole Grain" stamps to food producers to use on their packaging to enable the consumer to easily identify foods containing whole grains. To receive a stamp, a product must have 8 grams of whole grains. If you see the "100%" stamp on a package, this means that all the grain in that product is whole and that the product contains at least 16 grams of whole grain per serving.

3. Stressful situations (why you overate, such as whether you were bored, lonely, or had problems).
4. How you felt after overeating.
5. All positive thoughts!

After a few days, you will start to see a pattern of your eating habits and stressful triggers to try to avoid.

CORRECT PORTION SIZES

Understanding how to eyeball correct portions will eventually become second nature. Unfortunately, we all have fallen prey to portion distortion, as portions in restaurants have doubled over the past few decades. We often don't listen to our bodies and ignore the signals of feeling full, then proceed to eat every morsel on our plate. Calorie counting is just not practical, but understanding what your food plate should look like and the correct size of portions will help you eat a well-balanced diet, enabling you to lose weight. The following visuals are an easy reference, but I recommend that you also use measuring cups, spoons, and a scale at first. These will be your new best friends.

- Tennis ball = 1 fruit serving
- Cassette tape = 1 slice bread, pre-sliced (1 serving of grain)
- Computer mouse = 4-oz. serving of uncooked meat or fish (4 servings of protein)
- 1 yogurt container = 8 oz. (1 serving of dairy)
- 1 baseball = 1 cup raw vegetables (1 serving of veggies)
- ½ baseball = ½ cup of cooked vegetables (1 serving of veggies)
- 9-volt battery = 1 fat serving or 1 oz. of cheese (1 dairy)

Quick Hand Visuals

- 2 fists = 1 cup
- 1 fist = ½ cup
- Palm of your hand = 3 oz. (a cooked serving of meat, or 3 proteins)
- Thumb = 1 oz. (a piece of cheese)

BUSY SUPER FIT MAMA'S ON-THE-GO FOODS

Time is a rare commodity when you're a mom, so have nutritious snacks at hand to keep yourself from straying from your healthy eating plan. The first step is to toss out junk food, and the next is to make a shopping

TRACEY'S SNACK CHOICES RANGING BETWEEN 100 AND 200 CALORIES

1 cup carrot strips with 2 tablespoons hummus and 4 whole-grain crackers (such as Triscuits)

Stonyfield Farm Organic YoCalcium yogurt served with a cup of carrots, celery, or raw broccoli for dipping

4 graham cracker squares spread with 1 tablespoon of natural peanut or almond butter

1 low-fat string cheese with two whole-grain crackers

1 cup fat-free skim milk blended with 1 cup fresh strawberries and ½ cup low-fat vanilla yogurt

1 Laughing Cow light cheese with three whole-grain crackers

1 cup of fruit topped with ¾ cup of low-fat yogurt sprinkled with Granola for crunch

1 Stonyfield Farm Light Smoothie

1 cup low-fat or light yogurt

1 hard-boiled egg dipped in 1 tablespoon light ranch dressing

1 large stalk celery stuffed with 1 tablespoon peanut butter

1 slice whole-wheat bread with 1 oz. turkey breast and mustard

1 hard-boiled organic omega-3 egg with one piece of toasted whole-grain bread

1 oz. reduced-fat cheese rolled in 2 oz. deli turkey or chicken meat

1 4-inch whole-wheat pita with 2 tablespoons hummus

½ cup low-fat cottage cheese with 1 cup sliced strawberries (or any kind of berries)

1 apple with 1 tablespoon peanut or almond butter

Raw vegetables (especially broccoli, celery, carrots, cauliflower, and red peppers) dipped in hummus

½ cup steamed soybeans (edamame)

Energy bars (Remember, you don't have to eat a whole energy bar at once; you can space one out, eating half in the morning and half in the afternoon, depending on your portion requirements for the day. My favorites are the Bellybar [see www.nutrabella.com], which has essential vitamins and minerals for women during and after pregnancy; Larabars [see www.larabar.com]; and the PowerBar Pria Nutrition Bar [see www.powerbar.com].)

1 bag Kellogg's All-Bran Snack Bites

1 bag Frito-Lay 100-Calorie Mini Bite Sun Chips

11 Stacy's Whole Wheat Bagel Chips

1 100-calorie packet of Wheat Thins

½ oz. baked tortilla chips with 2 tablespoons salsa

20 animal crackers

3 to 4 cups of microwavable popcorn (make sure it has no more than 120 calories and 3 grams of fat)

7 Whole Wheat Triscuits

1–2 cups low-sodium (less than 350 milligrams) chicken noodle soup with 2 saltine crackers

10 almonds

10 cashews

½ cup Breyers All Natural Strawberry Ice Cream

½ cup Stonyfield Farm Organic Frozen Yogurt

list (see below for a few items to put on your shopping list, and be sure to read Chapter 11, too, before you go gathering). When you go grocery shopping, stick to the list.

One more word of advice: Don't go food shopping when you're hungry, otherwise a few extra goodies will make their way into the cart. Unfortunately, eating healthy and nutritiously does require a little preparation and thought, but with a little practice you will eventually get your system for success down. Here are some must-have Super Mama food staples. Make sure you have plenty of the following foods on hand for when the munchies strike:

Low-fat (organic) string cheese

Whole-wheat crackers

Whole-wheat bread

Natural peanut butter or other nut butters

Nuts and seeds (measure ¼ cup servings into bags to control portion size; this is equal to 1 serving of fat)

Fruit selection (preferably organic)

Low-fat (organic) yogurt (look for choices with high calcium content, including Greek yogurt and yogurt drinks or kefir)

Free-range organic omega-3-enriched eggs (pre-boil the eggs—they make a great 70-calorie nutritious snack)

Amy's Kitchen (www.amys.com) has some wonderful pre-packaged meals that are fabulous when you just don't feel like cooking or you're looking for a fuss-free nutritious lunch or dinner. What I love about Amy's foods is that they're made from organic produce and whole grains without any additives. Here are just a few of my favorite Amy's meals:

Brown Rice, Black Eyed Peas & Veggie Bowl

Tofu Scramble in a Pocket Sandwich

Quarter Pound Veggie Burgers

Organic Family Marinara Sauce

Low Fat Vegetable Barley Soup

Low Fat Black Bean Vegetable Soup

Low Fat Split Pea Soup

Fat Free Chunky Vegetable Soup

Success Story

....

Dariela Cruz, 37, North Hollywood, CA

Lost

15 lbs

3 sizes

11 Inches

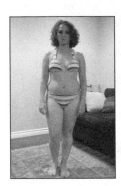 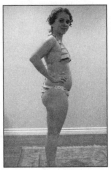 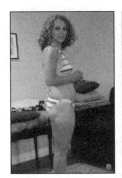 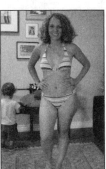

Before   After

• • • • •

Frustrated that her clothes were too tight and that she'd have to start buying bigger sizes, Dariela longed for her pre-baby body. The problem? She was unsure how to get it back. When she heard about Super Fit Mama, she felt like her prayers were answered. "The fact that it was a program that combines a food plan and workouts especially made for moms really attracted me," she says. "In the past, I've tried to exercise and eat healthy, but didn't get results. With Super Fit Mama, I didn't have to think about anything except following the plan and saw changes in my body quickly." The latter was extremely motivating.

Dariela especially loved that the workouts were short enough to squeeze into her day—at some point. "A few times when I couldn't wake up in the morning to exercise like I planned, I could easily do them at night and actually felt energized," Dariela says. "Plus, as I saw changes in my body it was easier to do the workouts because I'd remind myself that I look better every time I do them." That realization came early. Within just a matter of weeks, Dariela's ab muscles began to show and she felt stronger than ever. "I realized that even doing daily things like carrying my son, diaper bag, laptop bag, and groceries were easier than before," she says. "I even started purposely parking my car far from the store entrance. Instead of being mad about not finding a closer spot, I was happy because I was getting exercise."

One of the most pleasantly surprising parts of the program was that Dariela could lose weight *and* feed her huge sweet tooth. "It was hard at first, but I discovered that I can get by with a lot less sugar and that fruit can satisfy my sugar cravings instead of the cookies and cakes that I used to eat," she says. "Also, I was thrilled when just a few weeks in I no longer felt that mid-day energy slump." Dariela was also amazed at how easy it was to stop drinking high-sugar, high-calorie juices. She traded these unhealthy drinks for sugar-free lightly flavored waters, caffeine and sugar-free iced tea, and plain water garnished with a few wedges of lemon or orange.

Shortly after she started Super Fit Mama, the compliments from friends and family came pouring in. "They kept saying that I was getting skinnier and looked amazing!" she says. But the biggest sense of pride comes from within herself. "This is the first time in my life that I've followed an eating and exercise routine for more than a week. What I love about the Super Fit Mama plan is that it's something you can use for the rest of your life. It's not a diet, but an easy lifestyle change that I feel so lucky to have found!" Even better than that realization is the one that "you can have a baby *and* feel sexy!"

MOTIVATION FROM TEAM MALLETT

"It took me a couple days to get used to the portions, but soon enough my stomach shrank. Now when I eat a meal, I am absolutely stuffed on the right sized portions! I wonder now how did I ever scarf down four times as much food! What an oinker I was!" —Erica Shepherd

"Writing down what I eat in my food log keeps me on track. I make sure to take a piece of paper in my purse wherever I go and write down what I ate right after I eat it. That is so helpful!" —Dariela Cruz

CHAPTER 11

SUPER FIT
MAMA MEALS

REMEMBER THE DAYS WHEN "HEALTHY EATING" MEANT YOU ATE foods fit for a rabbit? Or when dieting meant you had to trade anything that actually tasted good for foods that tasted like cardboard? Well, times have changed. I am a real woman and a real mom. I also love food and am not going to settle for a life of naked salads or live in a bland, no-fat, no fun world. As a result, I've spent a lot of time over the years researching ways to make healthy foods that are delicious and highly nutritious. In fact, they're so delicious that my kids don't have a clue that they're good for them (and I plan to keep it that way!).

The following are some of my favorite recipes, but to make sure that they had all the important nutrients that both moms-to-be and new moms need, I consulted with Ivy Larson, mother of one and author of *The Whole Foods Diet Cookbook*. We made sure to include recipes that are low in fat and high in fiber since foods like these are a huge key to slimming down and keeping the weight off. What I love about each and every one of the twenty-five recipes here is that, while they're jam-packed with essential vitamins and minerals, they're also jam-packed with taste.

Another top criteria for the recipes I'd include was time. If you can't make it in under 30 minutes, it didn't make the cut. After all, whether you're a busy pregnant (and ravenous) woman or a new mom trying to juggle and adjust to your new life, you simply don't have much time to spend in the kitchen. (And with an adorable, new baby to love and hug, who wants to?) Plus, now that you're a mom (or going to be one shortly), you're no longer cooking just for yourself. You're cooking for your family. My children notice my eating habits all the time. If I have a piece of chocolate, so do they; if I take a sip of soda, so do they. I promise that if you start with healthy eating habits now, you'll be very glad later.

Here are a few tips to help out in the kitchen when you have a busy life:

1. Double the amount of the ingredients each time you cook a meal and then freeze the rest. This way when time is tight and you're in a rush, you'll have a healthy meal on hand. Just make sure you jot the date down on the freezer bag or container so you know how long the frozen meals will stay fresh.

2. If you don't like to freeze meals ahead, you can cut down on daily prep time by preparing some ingredients for the week ahead of time. For example, you can chop veggies in advance and store them in the refrigerator, or chop up meats ahead of time. (But be sure not to use the same utensils and cutting board with veggies after cutting your meats without a thorough washing.)

3. Invest in a slow cooker—they're awesome for making healthy stews, chili, and endless recipes while you're caring for your children. One of my favorite slow cooker recipe books is *Cooking Light Slow Cooker*.

4. Get a rice cooker for cooking whole grains. Rice cookers are not just for rice; they can be used for just about any whole grain. All you have to do is measure the water and the grain—and once cooked, they'll last three or four days in a covered container in your refrigerator. This will allow you to do something different with them each night. For example, if you make millet in the rice cooker, you can add it to soup, chili, or stew on night one, make a millet pilaf on night two, and so on.

5. Shop just once a week and plan menus in advance. If you know what you're going to make ahead of time, meal prep is much faster and easier.

6. Organizing and cleaning the kitchen will go a long way toward making meal prep faster. Organize your spices (toss the old ones), put canned goods in one spot, pastas and rice in another, and so on. Then clean the refrigerator out once a week and clean the freezer out once every two weeks.

When possible, opt for organic ingredients. However, I know that's not always feasible due to cost and availability. So if a recipe calls for an organic item, it's okay to substitute one that isn't.

Here's a snapshot of the recipes:

BREAKFAST:

- Lemony Flax Pancakes with Fresh Strawberries
- "Whey Healthy" Smoothie, 2 Ways
- Apple-n-Date Breakfast Bread Pudding
- Cinnamon Ricotta-Oatmeal Pancakes
- Southwest Breakfast Scramble
- Grab-n-Go Protein-Rich Lemony Cereal "Cookies"
- Peach and Almond Smoothie

LUNCH:

- Whole-Grain Pesto Pita Pizza with Fresh Tomatoes, Basil, and Ricotta
- Chicken Caesar Salad–Stuffed Sprouted Corn Tortillas
- Express-Style Garbanzo Bean and Fire-Roasted Tomato Soup
- Italian-Style Bread and Tuna Salad
- Curried Chicken and Green Grape Salad
- Mediterrancan Pasta Salad with Kalamata Olives, Red Peppers, and Rotisserie Chicken (or Tuna)
- Broccoli, Turkey, and Cheese Wrap

DINNER:

- Classic Vegetable and Beef Stew
- Black Bean, Sweet Potato, and Turkey Chili
- Tofu Provencal
- Effortless Veggie Lover's Lasagna
- Chicken Nuggets, Corn on the Cob, and Cream of Spinach Soup
- Roasted Vegetable Salad with Yogurt-Marinated Chicken and Garlic-Lime Vinaigrette
- Fiesta Salmon (or Turkey!) Burgers with a Side of Artichoke, Spinach, and Tomato Salad

DESSERT:

- Creamy Mango-Raspberry Freeze
- Spiced Pumpkin Custard with Caramel Sauce
- Honey-Roasted Peaches Topped with Lemony Cream
- Grilled Pineapple Kabobs with Easy Fruit Dip

BREAKFAST

LEMONY FLAX PANCAKES WITH FRESH STRAWBERRIES

Serves: 1

Who says pancakes can't be healthy? These almost flourless pancakes are super rich in those good-for-you omega-3 essential fatty acids and tummy-filling fiber and they're full of flavor too! Even better, they can be made in minutes. Consider doubling or tripling the recipe to serve the kids, or make ahead and refrigerate for the next day.

1 egg, lightly beaten (omega-3 organic egg, if possible)
¼ cup plain unsweetened soy milk (such as Silk)
2 tablespoons water
¼ teaspoon pure lemon extract
1 tablespoon ground flaxseeds (such as Barlean's)
2 tablespoons wheat germ
2 tablespoons white whole-wheat flour (or whole-wheat pastry flour)
Pinch of salt
1 teaspoon organic extra virgin coconut oil (such as Barlean's)
½ cup fresh strawberries, sliced

1. In a small bowl, whisk the egg, soy milk, water, and lemon extract together. Add the flaxseeds, wheat germ, flour, and pinch of salt. Mix to combine.
2. Heat the extra virgin coconut oil in a medium non-stick skillet over medium-high heat. Ladle out one-third of the batter and cook about 1 minute, or until edges easily lift. Flip and cook for an additional 1–2 minutes. Repeat with the remaining batter (you should end up with three pancakes). Serve pancakes with fresh strawberries on top.

FOOD EXCHANGES PER SERVING: 1 PROTEIN, ¼ DAIRY, 1 FRUIT, ½ GRAIN, 2 FAT

"WHEY HEALTHY" SMOOTHIE, 2 WAYS

Serves: 1

Both varieties of this nutritious breakfast smoothie are sure to give you plenty of zip, pep, and go! By using frozen fruit it gives the smoothie a creamy milkshake-like richness and subtle sweetness—but with no added sugar and no added fat! It's perfect before your next morning workout. The whey protein is a super-healthy lean protein source that not only helps build muscle and burn fat, but also helps your immune system function properly and even enhances your recovery time between workouts. The flaxseeds provide essential omega-3 fatty acids plus lots of fiber.

Smoothie 1: Mango-Lemon
1 scoop vanilla whey protein
1 cup frozen mango chunks
¾ cup low-fat organic, plain yogurt
1½ teaspoons pure lemon extract
1 tablespoon ground flaxseeds (such as Barlean's)

1. Place all ingredients in a blender; process until smooth and creamy. Drink at once.

FOOD EXCHANGES PER SERVING: 1 PROTEIN, 1 DAIRY, 2 FRUIT, 1 FAT

Smoothie 2: Cherry-Almond
1 scoop vanilla whey protein
1 cup frozen pitted cherries
¾ cup low-fat organic, plain yogurt
1½ teaspoons pure almond extract
1 tablespoon ground flaxseeds (such as Barlean's)

1. Place all ingredients in a blender; process until smooth and creamy. Drink at once.

FOOD EXCHANGES PER SERVING: 1 PROTEIN, 1 DAIRY, 2 FRUIT, 1 FAT

APPLE-N-DATE BREAKFAST BREAD PUDDING

Serves: 6

If you love bread pudding, you're in for a real treat with this deceptively nutritious breakfast casserole, which has all the yummy goodness of the dessert version, but without the added sugar and fat. In fact, there's just 3 tablespoons of sugar in the *whole* thing! It's still sweet and rich tasting though, thanks to the naturally sweet dates and apples. The spices further intensify the natural sweetness of the fruit. Best of all, you can make it ahead, keep it in the fridge, and enjoy a delicious fast-food breakfast for several days in a row.

1 teaspoon organic butter

3 large apples, chopped (keep the skins on!)

¾ cup chopped dates

1 teaspoon cinnamon, plus more to taste

¼ teaspoon nutmeg

2 tablespoons water

4 slices sprouted whole-grain bread (such as Food for Life Ezekiel 4:9 bread), torn into bite-sized pieces

3 tablespoons brown sugar, divided

4 eggs (omega-3 organic eggs, if possible)

1 cup low-fat milk

1 teaspoon pure vanilla extract

1. Heat the oven to 350 degrees. Spray an 8 x 8–inch baking dish with canola oil cooking spray.
2. Melt butter in a large non-stick skillet over medium-high heat. Add apples and dates. Sprinkle with 1 teaspoon cinnamon and measured nutmeg. Add the water. Cook for about 8 minutes, or until apples are soft but not mushy. Set aside.
3. Arrange the bread pieces on the bottom of the prepared baking dish. Sprinkle with 1 tablespoon brown sugar plus cinnamon to taste. Spread the apple-date mixture on top.
4. In a small bowl, whisk together the eggs, milk, vanilla extract, and remaining 2 tablespoons of brown sugar. Pour custard mixture on top of apples.
5. Bake for 50–55 minutes. Remove casserole from oven and let sit 10 minutes before serving. Serve warm.

FOOD EXCHANGES FOR 1 SERVING: 1 DAIRY, 1 FRUIT, 1 GRAIN

CINNAMON RICOTTA-OATMEAL PANCAKES

Serves: 1

These almost flourless pancakes are loaded with fiber-rich whole-grain oats. They also pack a powerful protein punch that will help keep you feeling full all morning long!

2 egg whites, slightly beaten (from omega-3 organic eggs, if possible)
¼ cup low-fat ricotta cheese
3 tablespoons water
2 tablespoons white whole-wheat flour (such as King Arthur brand)
¼ cup old-fashioned oats (such as Quaker Old Fashioned Oats)
½ teaspoon cinnamon, plus more to taste
¼ teaspoon allspice
⅛ teaspoon pure almond extract
2 teaspoons molasses, divided
Dash of salt
Canola oil cooking spray
½ Granny Smith apple, chopped

1. In a small bowl, whisk together the egg whites, ricotta, and water. Add the flour, oatmeal, cinnamon, allspice, almond extract, 1 teaspoon of molasses, and dash of salt. Mix well to thoroughly combine ingredients.
2. Spray a large non-stick skillet with canola oil cooking spray. Ladle batter onto hot skillet to form 4 equal small pancakes. Cook about 1 minute per side, or until edges easily lift. Flip and cook for an additional 1–2 minutes, or until cooked through. Transfer pancakes to a plate.
3. Place chopped apple, remaining teaspoon of molasses, and cinnamon to taste in a microwave-safe dish. Heat on high for 1½ minutes. Top pancakes with apples and serve.

FOOD EXCHANGES PER SERVING: 1 PROTEIN, 1 DAIRY, 1 FRUIT, 3 GRAINS

SOUTHWEST BREAKFAST SCRAMBLE

Serves: 1

Here's the ideal morning jump-start recipe to help you sneak tofu in under the radar. When you scramble extra-firm tofu with an egg, the tofu becomes completely irresistible.

1 teaspoon extra virgin olive oil
¼ cup diced red onions
½ red bell pepper, diced
1 egg (omega-3 organic egg, if possible)
¼ cup crumbled extra-firm tofu, drained and patted as dry as possible with paper towels
¼ cup prepared salsa
2 tablespoons shredded organic low-fat cheddar cheese
⅓ cup black beans, rinsed and drained
⅛ teaspoon cumin
Pinch of cayenne pepper
Salt, to taste

1. Heat the extra virgin olive oil in a large non-stick skillet over medium-high heat. Add onion and bell pepper and sauté 5–6 minutes, or until vegetables are soft.
2. In a medium-sized bowl, whisk the egg, tofu, salsa, and cheddar cheese together. Add the black beans, cumin, pinch of cayenne, and salt to taste.
3. Pour the egg and bean mixture over the sautéed vegetables. Scramble over medium-high heat until eggs are cooked through. Eat at once.

FOOD EXCHANGES PER SERVING: 1.5 PROTEIN, 1 DAIRY, 1 VEGGIE, 1 GRAIN, 1 FAT

GRAB-N-GO PROTEIN-RICH LEMONY CEREAL "COOKIES"

Yields 12 servings
Here's a fun, delicious, and creative way to eat your cereal on the run.
These grab-n-go cereal "cookies" are great with a glass of soy milk or
low-fat organic milk. P.S. These are perfect for kids and a nutritious alternative to sugar-laden granola bars.

2 cups cornflakes (such as Nature's Path)
⅔ cup white whole-wheat flour (such as King Arthur brand)
½ teaspoon baking soda
½ teaspoon salt
1 teaspoon orange zest (available in the spice section of your supermarket, such as Spice Islands brand)
¼ cup brown sugar
3 tablespoons ground flaxseeds (such as Barlean's)
1 egg, lightly beaten (omega-3 organic egg, if possible)
¼ cup canola oil
2 teaspoons pure lemon extract
¾ cup organic low-fat small-curd cottage cheese

1. Preheat oven to 400 degrees. Spray a baking sheet with canola oil
   cooking spray.
2. Place cornflakes in a blender or food processor and pulse into fine
   crumbs. Add cornflake crumbs to a medium-sized bowl; mix in flour,
   baking soda, salt, orange zest, sugar, and flaxseeds.
3. In a separate bowl, mix together the egg, oil, lemon extract, and
   cottage cheese. Add the dry ingredients to the wet ingredients and
   mix until just moistened.
4. Drop about 2 tablespoons of batter per cookie onto the baking sheet.
   Flatten the batter with the back of a fork. Bake cookies for about
   15 minutes. Remove cookies from oven and let cool and harden for
   10 minutes before eating.

FOOD EXCHANGES PER COOKIE: 1 GRAIN, 1 FAT

PEACH AND ALMOND SMOOTHIE

Serves: 1

Smoothies are a delicious and convenient way to introduce (or sneak!) nutrient-rich tofu into your diet. This creamy and rich-tasting breakfast takes less than 5 minutes to prepare, so it's ideal for those crazy busy mornings when you barely have time to get dressed! The great thing about smoothies is that you can put them in a thermos and drink them while you drive to work—or wherever it is you go.

½ cup low-fat organic milk or plain unsweetened soy milk (such as Silk)
4 ounces silken tofu (about ¼ package of Nasoya brand Silken Tofu)
¾ cup frozen peaches
2 teaspoons almond butter
1 teaspoon pure almond extract
1 teaspoon raw honey (optional)

1. Combine all ingredients in a blender and process for 1 minute, or until smooth and creamy. Enjoy at once.

FOOD EXCHANGES PER SERVING: 1½ PROTEIN, ½ DAIRY, 1 FRUIT, 1 FAT

LUNCH

WHOLE-GRAIN PESTO PITA PIZZA WITH FRESH TOMATOES, BASIL, AND RICOTTA

Serves: 1

Not much can satisfy a nagging, gnawing hard-core pizza craving when it hits! Now you can satisfy your craving and still optimize nutrition without blowing your diet with this fiber-rich and delish healthy version. Best of all, you can prepare this faster than you can dial take-out.

1 6-inch oat bran pita (such as Toufayan brand), carefully cut in half so that you have 2 very thin round pieces
1 tablespoon prepared pesto
1 firm tomato, cut into very thin rounds
Salt, to taste
Garlic powder, to taste
Freshly ground black pepper, to taste
2 tablespoons low-fat organic ricotta cheese
Drizzle of extra virgin olive oil
1 tablespoon chopped fresh basil
⅓ cup shredded low-fat organic mozzarella cheese

1. Preheat oven to 400 degrees. Spray a large non-stick baking sheet with extra virgin olive oil cooking spray. Place the two pita rounds on the baking sheet.
2. Spread the pesto over each pita. Arrange the tomato slices on top of the pitas. Season tomatoes with salt, garlic powder, and pepper to taste. Spread the ricotta cheese on top of the seasoned tomatoes. Bake pizzas for 8 minutes.
3. Remove pizzas from the oven. Sprinkle with fresh basil. Top pizzas with mozzarella. Bake for an additional 2–3 minutes, or until mozzarella melts. Eat at once!

FOOD EXCHANGES PER SERVING: 3 PROTEIN, 1 VEGGIE, 1 GRAIN, 1 FAT

CHICKEN CAESAR SALAD–STUFFED SPROUTED CORN TORTILLAS

Serves: 1

If you always seem to find leftover chicken breasts or a half-eaten rotisserie chicken sitting in your fridge, here's the perfect express-lane midday meal to satisfy your hunger. I've included a great Caesar recipe below using flaxseed oil, but you can always choose a high-quality prepared dressing if you like (I particularly love Annie's Naturals brand). If you choose to make my Caesar dressing, you'll certainly have leftovers, but you can always serve the rest for dinner (if you aren't in the mood for another lettuce-based salad, try drizzling the Caesar over steamed and chilled chopped asparagus for a delicious lettuce-free salad). *(Note: There will probably be more than enough dressing; leftovers can be stored in a covered container in the refrigerator for up to two days.)*

Caesar Dressing:
1 or 2 anchovy fillets, mashed with a fork (optional)
¼ cup low-fat plain Greek-style yogurt
2 teaspoons crushed garlic
1 tablespoon canola-oil mayonnaise (such as Hellmann's)
1 teaspoon lemon juice
1 teaspoon Dijon mustard
1 teaspoon Worcestershire sauce

1. In a medium-sized bowl, add the mashed anchovies (if using), yogurt, garlic, mayonnaise, lemon juice, Dijon mustard, and Worcestershire sauce. Whisk until smooth.

FOOD EXCHANGES PER SERVING: 1 PROTEIN, 3 FAT

Tortillas:
¼ cup chopped cooked chicken (either chicken breast or rotisserie chicken)
1 cup Romaine lettuce, finely chopped
2 tablespoons shaved Parmesan cheese
¼ cup cherry tomatoes, cut into halves lengthwise
2 tablespoons sliced black olives

Salt, to taste

Freshly ground black pepper, to taste

1 tablespoon Caesar dressing (recipe above or prepared all-natural brand, such as Annie's Naturals)

2 sprouted corn tortillas (such as Food for Life brand)

Extra virgin olive oil cooking spray

Hot sauce, to taste (optional)

1. Combine chopped cooked chicken and Romaine lettuce in a large bowl. Add the Parmesan, cherry tomatoes, and olives. Season with salt and pepper to taste. Add 1 tablespoon prepared Caesar dressing (such as Annie's Naturals) or recipe (above). Toss salad ingredients together.

2. Spray a large cast iron skillet or non-stick skillet with extra virgin olive oil cooking spray; heat over medium-high. When skillet is hot, add tortillas and cook about 2–3 minutes per side.

3. Pile tossed chicken Caesar salad equally on top of each heated tortilla; fold tortillas in half. Drizzle with hot sauce (optional). Eat at once!

FOOD EXCHANGES PER SERVING: 2 PROTEIN, 1 VEGGIE, 2 GRAINS, ½ FAT

EXPRESS-STYLE GARBANZO BEAN AND FIRE-ROASTED TOMATO SOUP

Serves: 2

Bean-based soups are such a satisfying, filling, and fiber-rich food, perfect for lunch! The problem is most bean soup recipes aren't exactly made express-lane style. Here, by using canned garbanzo beans and canned fire-roasted tomatoes you'll still get great depth of flavor without the time commitment. The soup only requires about 8 minutes of hands-on time. Let it simmer just 10 minutes while you feed the kids. This recipe serves two, so make it on a playdate day and share with a friend or save the rest for leftovers. *(Note: The soup will keep for up to three days if stored in a covered container in the refrigerator.)*

2 tablespoons extra virgin olive oil
5 cloves chopped garlic
1 large Spanish onion, chopped
1 teaspoon cumin
Salt, to taste
1 can (14.5 ounces) fire-roasted diced tomatoes (such as Muir Glen brand)
1 cup all-natural vegetable broth (such as Imagine Organic brand)
1 can (15 ounces) garbanzo beans, rinsed and drained
¼ cup shaved Parmesan cheese, divided

1. Heat extra virgin olive oil in a large saucepan over medium-high heat. Add garlic and onion and sauté about 5–6 minutes. Season with cumin and salt to taste. Add fire-roasted tomatoes and cook 2–3 minutes. Add vegetable broth and garbanzo beans. Simmer, uncovered, for 10 minutes.
2. Remove about 1½ cups of soup, mostly beans, and set aside to cool. Transfer cooled bean mixture to a blender and process until smooth but still somewhat chunky. Pour pureed bean mixture back with the remainder of the soup. Heat for 1 minute. Serve warm with Parmesan cheese on top.

FOOD EXCHANGES PER SERVING: 1 PROTEIN, ½ DAIRY, 1 VEGGIE, 2½ GRAINS, 3 FAT

ITALIAN-STYLE BREAD AND TUNA SALAD

Serves: 1

This no-cook main-dish rustic and easy-to-assemble salad is perfect for a Tuscan-inspired lunch break. Called *panzanella*, most Italian-style bread salads use white day-old crusty bread, but this super healthy version calls for sprouted whole-grain bread instead. You'll get a lot more fiber and significantly more nutrients by using whole-grain bread and you'll feel substantially more full and satisfied throughout the afternoon. You might not even need a snack . . .

1 teaspoons extra virgin olive oil
1 teaspoon crushed garlic
1 slice sprouted whole-grain bread (such as Food for Life Ezekiel 4:9 bread)
Salt, to taste
Freshly ground black pepper, to taste
1 firm tomato, coarsely chopped
¼ cup finely chopped red onion
½ cucumber, peeled, seeded, and chopped
2 tablespoons chopped fresh basil
3 ounces water-packed canned tuna, flaked
1 teaspoon flaxseed oil (such as Barlean's)
2 teaspoons balsamic vinegar

1. Heat extra virgin olive oil in a large non-stick skillet over medium-high heat. Add garlic and sauté 30 seconds. Add bread pieces and season with salt and pepper to taste. Toast bread cubes, stirring frequently, for 4–5 minutes. Set aside.
2. In a medium-sized serving dish, add tomato, red onion, cucumber, basil, and tuna. Add the bread and toss. Drizzle with flaxseed oil and balsamic vinegar. Season with salt and pepper to taste. For the best flavor, let salad sit 30 minutes before eating.

FOOD EXCHANGES PER SERVING: 3 PROTEIN, 1 VEGGIE, 1 GRAIN, 2 FAT

CURRIED CHICKEN AND GREEN GRAPE SALAD

Serves: 1

This easy recipe may well become one of your favorite go-to everyday 15-minute lunches. It's the curry that really takes the flavor over the top. Feel free to double, triple, or quadruple the recipe and serve to the whole family! Also, if you can't do chicken, feel free to substitute 4 ounces of extra-firm tofu, drained, patted as dry as possible with paper towels, and cut into 1 x ½–inch portions (1 protein food exchange). *(Note: This salad will keep for 24 hours in the refrigerator in a covered container.)*

¼ cup chopped pecans

1 teaspoon curry powder

1 tablespoon whole-wheat flour or white whole-wheat flour (such as King Arthur brand)

3 ounces boneless, skinless chicken breasts cut into cubes

1 teaspoon extra virgin olive oil

¼ cup thinly sliced celery

1 heaping tablespoon minced onion

⅓ cup pre-cut matchstick carrots

1 cup green grapes, halved

1 tablespoon dried cranberries

2 heaping tablespoons organic fat-free Greek yogurt (such as Fage)

1 tablespoon reduced-fat sour cream

⅛ teaspoon salt

Several Bibb lettuce leaves

1. Preheat oven to 400 degrees.
2. Coarsely chop pecans and spread on cookie sheet; toast in the oven for about 10 minutes.
3. Meanwhile, add curry and flour to a zip-top bag and shake to mix. Add chicken cubes to the bag and shake to coat chicken in the curry and flour.
4. Heat the oil in a large non-stick skillet over medium heat, tilting the skillet to spread the oil evenly. Add chicken to the hot skillet and cook for 3–5 minutes each side. Remove chicken with a spatula and set on paper towels to drain and cool.
5. In a large bowl, mix together celery, onion, carrots, toasted pecans, sliced grapes, dried cranberries, and chicken. In a separate bowl, mix together the yogurt, low-fat sour cream, and salt; add to the other ingredients and toss gently. Dish salad onto lettuce leaves and eat!

FOOD EXCHANGES PER SERVING: 3 PROTEIN, ½ DAIRY, 2½ FRUIT, 4½ FAT

MEDITERRANEAN PASTA SALAD WITH KALAMATA OLIVES, RED PEPPERS, AND ROTISSERIE CHICKEN (OR TUNA)

Serves: 1

Unlike most salads, this slightly spicy Mediterranean-inspired and easy-to-prepare lunch entrée is extremely satisfying and filling. Although it's low in fat (thanks to swapping rich and creamy Greek yogurt for high-fat mayonnaise), your tastebuds won't suspect a thing! The plump and juicy kalamata olives and sweet, fragrant fresh basil add a touch of gourmet splash, while the red pepper flakes add just a speck of heat.

1 cup of *cooked* whole-wheat rigatoni
1 red bell pepper, diced
5 kalamata olives, minced
2 ounces chopped rotisserie chicken (or water-packed canned tuna, drained and crumbled)
¼ teaspoon Dijon mustard
½ teaspoon flaxseed oil (such as Barlean's)
1 teaspoon balsamic vinegar
1 tablespoon fat-free Greek yogurt (such as Fage)
Salt, to taste
Red pepper flakes, to taste
¼ cup chopped fresh basil
1 tablespoon crumbled low-fat feta cheese

1. In a medium-sized bowl, toss the cooked rigatoni with the bell pepper, olives, and chicken.
2. In a small bowl, whisk together the mustard, flaxseed oil, balsamic vinegar, and yogurt. Add vinaigrette to pasta mixture and toss to combine.
3. Season pasta with salt and red pepper flakes to taste. Add basil and crumbled feta. Toss to combine. Let salad sit for 10 minutes before eating. Eat at room temperature.

FOOD EXCHANGES PER SERVING: 2 PROTEIN, 1 VEGGIE, 2 GRAINS, 1½ FAT

BROCCOLI, TURKEY, AND CHEESE WRAP

Serves: 1

Why pack up the kids and go on a deli run when you can easily make your own wrap in less than 10 minutes? Not only can this wrap be made in a hurry, it's way healthier and definitely tastier than that deli fix, thanks to minimal oil, extra veggies, and a whole-grain wrap.

1 sprouted whole-grain tortilla (such as Food for Life brand)
1 cup frozen broccoli florets
1 teaspoon extra virgin olive oil
1 clove minced garlic
¼ red bell pepper, finely chopped
¼ cup red onion, finely chopped
Old Bay Seasoning (available in the seasoning section of your
    supermarket), to taste
¼ cup shredded low-fat cheddar cheese
2 ounces chopped deli turkey

1. Preheat oven to 350 degrees. Wrap tortilla in foil and place in oven on a rack while you prepare the filling, warming the tortilla about 8–10 minutes.
2. Place the broccoli in a microwave-safe dish and heat on high for 2 minutes.
3. Heat the extra virgin olive oil in a small non-stick skillet over medium-high heat; add garlic, red bell pepper, and red onion. Sauté vegetables for 3–4 minutes, or until soft. Add broccoli florets. Season vegetables with Old Bay Seasoning to taste (a little goes a long way!). Add the cheese and turkey and cook, stirring constantly, until cheese melts.
4. Remove warm tortilla from the oven and transfer to a large plate. Place broccoli, cheese, and turkey filling on the tortilla near one edge, roll the tortilla, and eat at once!

FOOD EXCHANGES PER SERVING: 3 PROTEIN, 1½ VEGGIES, 1 GRAIN, 1 FAT

DINNER

CLASSIC VEGETABLE AND BEEF STEW

Serves: 4

This delish one-dish meal and perennial classic is brimming with fiber-rich veggies. The slight hint of orange updates the flavor and the extra-lean beef keeps the saturated fat to an absolute bare minimum. It calls for a Spanish onion, which is similar to a regular yellow onion but milder and sweeter. If your grocery store does not have Spanish onions, you can substitute any sweet onion.

1 tablespoon extra virgin olive oil
1 Spanish onion, chopped
4 cloves crushed garlic
1 pound lean beef stew meat, preferably from grass-fed beef (trimmed of all fat and cut into 1-inch cubes)
Salt, to taste
Freshly ground black pepper, to taste
Garlic powder, to taste
1 cup finely chopped carrots
3 tablespoons white whole-wheat flour (or regular whole-wheat flour)

3 cups vegetable broth (such as Imagine Organic brand)
1 can (14.5 ounces) diced tomatoes (such as Muir Glen brand)
1 teaspoon balsamic vinegar
2 tablespoons orange juice concentrate
4 fresh thyme sprigs, tied with kitchen twine
8 ounces sliced button mushrooms (buy pre-sliced to save time)
1½ cups frozen lima beans, thawed to room temperature
1½ cups frozen corn kernels, thawed to room temperature

1. Heat extra virgin olive oil in a large saucepan over medium-high heat. Add the onion and crushed garlic; sauté for 5–6 minutes. Season beef with salt, pepper, and garlic powder. Add beef to the saucepan and cook 4–5 minutes, or until mostly cooked through. Add carrots and cook an additional 3–4 minutes. Stir in flour and cook for 1 minute.

2. Add the vegetable broth, diced tomatoes, balsamic vinegar, orange juice concentrate, button mushrooms, and thyme sprigs. Cover and simmer for 15 minutes.

3. Add lima beans and corn. Cook, uncovered, for an additional 5 minutes. Serve warm.

FOOD EXCHANGES PER SERVING: 4 PROTEIN, 1½ VEGGIES, 2½ GRAINS, 1 FAT

BLACK BEAN, SWEET POTATO, AND TURKEY CHILI

Serves: 6

This intriguing, mildly sweet, and somewhat spicy twist on traditional chili commands attention! The subtle smokiness from the fire-roasted tomatoes combines beautifully with the natural sweetness of the sweet potatoes. The spiciness of three complementary seasonings—cumin, coriander, and cayenne—takes the flavor over the top. If your grocery store does not have Spanish onions, you may substitute any mild, sweet onion.

2 medium-sized sweet potatoes
2 tablespoons extra virgin olive oil
2 Spanish onions, chopped
5 cloves garlic, minced
Salt, to taste
1 pound extra-lean ground turkey
1 can (4.5 ounces) chopped green chiles
2 cans (15 ounces each) fire-roasted diced tomatoes
1 can (15 ounces) black beans, rinsed and drained
1 teaspoon cumin
1 teaspoon coriander
Cayenne pepper, to taste
¼ cup cilantro, chopped
½ cup crumbled coastal cheddar cheese (Coastal cheddar is a gourmet specialty white cheese that has little crunchy sea salt crystals added to it during the aging process. It has a full, savory flavor and crumbles easily. If you can't find coastal cheddar, you can substitute feta cheese

if you want a cheese that crumbles well or freshly shaved Parmesan if you want to more closely match the flavor.)

1. Use a fork to poke holes in the sweet potatoes. Bake sweet potatoes in a 400-degree oven for 1 hour or until done. Remove sweet potatoes from the oven and set aside to cool. When cool enough to handle, remove the skins and mash. Set mashed sweet potatoes aside.
2. Heat extra virgin olive oil in a large saucepan over medium-high heat. Add the chopped onion and garlic and sauté for 4–5 minutes, or until onion is soft. Season with salt and cayenne to taste. Add the ground turkey, season with additional salt, and cook until meat is no longer pink. Add the chopped green chiles, diced tomatoes, black beans, cumin, coriander, and cayenne pepper to taste (I use several pinches). Cook, uncovered, for 15 minutes. Ladle chili into serving bowls and garnish with cilantro and crumbled coastal cheddar cheese (optional).

FOOD EXCHANGES PER SERVING: 3 PROTEIN, 1½ VEGGIE, 1 GRAIN, 1 FAT

TOFU PROVENCAL

Serves: 4

The flavors in this dish are inspired from the region of Provence in southern France that borders the Mediterranean Sea. The fresh and flavorsome food traditionally eaten in Provence more resemble Italian, Greek, or Spanish cuisine than typical French fare. Admittedly they may not eat much tofu in southern France, but if you love food from this region and you're looking to add more tofu to your diet, this dish is tops. Also, even if you are not much of an anchovy fan, you definitely want to follow the recipe and keep the anchovy here as it adds a nutty rather than fishy flavor when sautéed with the oil, butter, and garlic. Finally, if you want an even heartier dish serve the tofu Provencal over sprouted whole-grain pasta tossed with a little extra virgin olive oil, salt, and oregano. It's also delicious served with a side of cannelloni beans.

1 block (14 ounces) extra-firm tofu

Salt, to taste

White pepper, to taste

1 egg, beaten (omega-3 organic egg, if possible)

¼ cup white whole-wheat flour (such as King Arthur brand)

½ teaspoon dried oregano

1 tablespoon plus 1 teaspoon extra virgin olive oil, divided

1 teaspoon organic butter

1 canned flat anchovy fillet, mashed with a fork

2 teaspoons minced garlic

2 small zucchini, sliced

Juice from 1 whole lemon

1 can (14.5 ounces) diced tomatoes

½ cup halved, pitted kalamata olives or other brine-cured black olives

1 tablespoon chopped fresh basil

1. Drain tofu and pat as dry as possible with paper towels. Cut tofu in half lengthwise. Cut both blocks in half down the middle, so you have four rectangular tofu cutlets. Season tofu cutlets with salt and white pepper.

2. Beat egg in a medium-sized bowl. Set aside. Mix flour and oregano together.

3. Pour 1 tablespoon extra virgin olive oil in a large non-stick skillet and heat over medium-high heat, tilting the skillet to evenly disperse the oil. While the oil heats, dip the tofu cutlets in the egg and then dredge in the flour mixture. Add the tofu cutlets and sear for about 4 minutes on each side, or until just golden brown. Remove the tofu cutlets with a slotted spoon and set them aside on a plate.

4. Add the remaining teaspoon of extra virgin olive oil and the butter to the "dirty" skillet; add mashed anchovy and garlic and cook about 30 seconds. Add zucchini and cook about 4 minutes. Season with salt to taste. Add the lemon juice and cook about 1 minute. Add the tomatoes and olives and cook 10–12 minutes, until most of the liquid has cooked off. Add tofu cutlets back to the skillet and cook 1 minute. Serve with chopped fresh basil on top.

FOOD EXCHANGES PER SERVING: 1 PROTEIN, ½ VEGGIE, ½ GRAIN, 1½ FAT

EFFORTLESS VEGGIE LOVER'S LASAGNA

Serves: 6

Seriously, does anyone not *love* lasagna? We can't think of too many people who wouldn't appreciate a delicious home-spun lasagna meal. Of course, if you're the one doing all the cooking, the big drawback is that most lasagna recipes require a hefty time commitment. Most aren't very healthy either. This dish solves both problems since: (1) it's very healthy (the tofu hides out amid the spinach, ricotta, and Parmesan), and (2) you don't have to pre-cook the noodles (the trick is to keep the noodles moist with marinara sauce while the lasagna is cooking). This is sure to become a family favorite!

2 boxes (10 ounces each) chopped frozen spinach, thawed, drained, and
    patted as dry as possible with paper towels
¾ cup low-fat ricotta cheese
¾ of a 14-ounce block of extra-firm tofu, drained, patted as dry as
    possible with paper towels, and crumbled
½ cup shredded Parmesan cheese
1 egg, lightly beaten (omega-3 organic egg, if possible)
2 teaspoons extra virgin olive oil
½ teaspoon salt
1 teaspoon garlic powder
1 teaspoon dried basil
2 jars (25 ounces each) marinara sauce (such as Rao's Homemade
    Marinara or Amy's Family Marinara), divided
9 whole-wheat lasagna noodles, uncooked
1 cup shredded low-fat organic mozzarella cheese

1. Preheat oven to 350 degrees.
2. In a large bowl, combine spinach, ricotta, crumbled tofu, Parmesan, egg, extra virgin olive oil, salt, garlic powder, and dried basil. Mix ingredients together thoroughly.
3. Spread 1 cup of marinara sauce on the bottom of a 9 x 13–inch baking dish. Arrange three noodles on top of the sauce. Spread ¾ cup marinara on top of the noodles. Spread half of the spinach-tofu mixture on top. Spread ½ cup marinara sauce on top, followed by three noodles and another ¾ cup of marinara. Spread the remaining half of the

spinach-tofu mixture on top, followed by ½ cup marinara, three more noodles, and another ¾ cup marinara. Sprinkle with mozzarella cheese. Cover dish with aluminum foil and bake for 40 minutes.

4. Uncover and bake for an additional 20 minutes. Remove lasagna from oven and let sit 15–20 minutes before serving.

FOOD EXCHANGES PER SERVING: 2 PROTEIN, ½ VEGGIE, 3 GRAINS, ½ FAT

CHICKEN NUGGETS, CORN ON THE COB, AND CREAM OF SPINACH SOUP

Serves: 4

This is one of those dinners your kids won't be able to get enough of. While most healthy chicken nuggets are a major disappointment, this recipe rocks! And, while I've found most kids won't go near spinach, the mild flavor and creaminess of spinach soup is the exception. Finally, the corn on the cob is easy to make and fun to eat . . . perfect for rounding out a well-balanced and nutritious family meal.

Chicken Nuggets:
½ cup whole-wheat panko crumbs (such as Ian's All-Natural brand available in supermarkets and at www.iansnaturalfoods.com)
1 cup cornflakes
¼ cup ground flaxseeds (such as Barlean's Forti-Flax)
2 tablespoons grated Parmesan cheese
½ teaspoon paprika
½ teaspoon garlic powder
1 teaspoon savory spice
1½ pounds boneless, skinless, free-range chicken breasts, cut into bite-sized nugget pieces
½ teaspoon salt
1 tablespoon extra virgin olive oil

1. Place the whole-wheat panko crumbs, cornflakes, flaxseeds, Parmesan, paprika, garlic powder, and savory in a food processor or blender; process into fine crumbs. Pour crumbs onto a large plate. Set aside.

2. Sprinkle ½ teaspoon of salt on chicken and toss to evenly distribute.

3. Roll chicken in the crumb mixture.

4. Heat the oil in a large non-stick skillet over medium-high heat. Place the chicken nuggets in the skillet in a single layer, being careful not to crowd the pan. Cook until golden and crispy on one side, about 3–4 minutes. Turn and cook on the other side until the chicken is cooked through and the coating is crisp and lightly browned. Serve warm.

FOOD EXCHANGES PER SERVING: 6 PROTEIN, 1 GRAIN, 1 FAT

Corn on the Cob:
4 ears fresh corn, husks removed
Flaxseed oil (such as Barlean's)
Salt, to taste
Freshly ground black pepper, to taste

1. Bring a large pot of salted water to a boil. Add corn and cook 5–6 minutes (or more if you like very tender corn). Carefully remove corn with a slotted spoon. Brush lightly with flaxseed oil. Season with salt and pepper to taste. Serve warm.

FOOD EXCHANGES PER SERVING: 2 GRAINS (FOR EACH EAR OF CORN)

Cream of Spinach Soup:
4 cups vegetable broth (such as Imagine Natural Foods)
1 tablespoon extra virgin olive oil
1 tablespoon butter
1 cup chopped Spanish onion (or any mild, sweet onion)
3 tablespoons white whole-wheat flour (such as King Arthur brand)
2 boxes (10 ounces each) frozen chopped spinach, thawed, drained, and patted as dry as possible with paper towels
⅛ teaspoon salt, plus more to taste
¼ teaspoon nutmeg
¼ teaspoon white pepper
½ cup silken tofu
½ cup low-fat milk (organic is preferable)

1. Pour vegetable broth into a small saucepan and heat over medium-high heat.
2. Melt oil and butter in a large saucepan over medium-high heat; add onions and sauté 5–6 minutes, or until soft. Whisk in flour and cook an additional minute. Add spinach, salt, nutmeg, and white pepper.
3. Pour warm vegetable broth into the saucepan with the spinach and onion mixture. Stir in the silken tofu and milk. Remove the saucepan from the heat. Working in small batches, ladle the mixture into a blender or food processor; process until smooth and creamy. Pour mixture back into the saucepan and heat over medium-high heat for 4–5 minutes, or until warmed through. Serve warm.

FOOD EXCHANGES PER SERVING: 1½ VEGGIE, 1 GRAIN, 1½ FAT

ROASTED VEGETABLE SALAD WITH YOGURT-MARINATED CHICKEN AND GARLIC-LIME VINAIGRETTE

Serves: 4

If you invite friends over for dinner, you surely don't want to serve them "diet" food—but you do still want to eat healthy yourself! Here's the perfect one-dish meal that won't have your friends dashing for a Big Mac as soon as they leave your house. As an added bonus, it's also effortlessly easy to make. The chicken, vinaigrette, and roasted veggies can all be prepared the day ahead, so all you have to do is assemble the salad right before your friends come. Oh! and it's even kid-friendly, since the little munchkins can just pick out the roasted carrots, potatoes, and chicken for a complete and balanced meal.

Yogurt Marinated Chicken:

1½ pounds boneless, skinless, free-range chicken, cut into bite-sized pieces

Salt, to taste

½ cup full-fat plain organic yogurt *(Note: Don't worry about using full-fat yogurt here since barely any of the yogurt actually stays on the chicken anyway! And, since the full-fat yogurt delivers far superior taste results compared to low-fat, it's worth using.)*

1 teaspoon cumin

1 teaspoon oregano

1 teaspoon garlic powder

½ teaspoon salt

2 tablespoon lime juice

Extra virgin olive oil cooking spray

1. Season chicken with salt.
2. In a large zip-top bag, combine the yogurt, cumin, oregano, garlic powder, salt, and lime juice. Mix ingredients well. Add chicken to the bag, transfer to the refrigerator, and marinate for at least 30 minutes (up to 4 hours is fine).
3. Remove the chicken from the marinade. Spray a large non-stick skillet with extra virgin olive oil cooking spray and heat over medium-high heat. Add chicken and cook 4–5 minutes on each side, or until cooked through. Remove the chicken from the skillet and set aside until you're ready to assemble the salad.

FOOD EXCHANGES PER SERVING: 6 PROTEIN

Garlic-Lime Vinaigrette:

2 tablespoons extra virgin olive oil

6 cloves chopped garlic

2 tablespoons lime juice

¼ teaspoon cumin

Salt, to taste

Freshly ground black pepper, to taste

1. Place oil, garlic, and lime juice in a microwave-safe bowl. Heat in microwave for 1½ minutes. Stir in cumin, salt, and pepper to taste. Set aside until ready to assemble salad.

FOOD EXCHANGES PER SERVING: 1½ FAT

Roasted Vegetable Salad:
1 eggplant, sliced into 1-inch thick rounds
1 tablespoon plus 1 teaspoon extra virgin olive oil, plus more for brushing
Salt, to taste
Freshly ground black pepper, to taste
1 large red onion, cut into 1-inch pieces
8 red-skinned potatoes, quartered
2 cups baby carrots
Cumin, to taste
Garlic powder, to taste
Oregano, to taste
5 ounces arugula leaves
½ cup chopped fresh basil
Freshly ground black pepper

1. Preheat broiler.
2. Brush both sides of eggplant with extra virgin olive oil. Season with salt and pepper to taste. Broil eggplant until just brown and just cooked through, about 2 minutes per side. Transfer eggplant slices to paper towels to drain. Set aside.
3. Preheat oven to 425 degrees.
4. Combine onions, potatoes, and carrots on a large foil-lined baking sheet. Toss vegetables with extra virgin olive oil, cumin, garlic powder, oregano, and salt to taste. Roast vegetables for 40 minutes. Remove vegetables from oven and set aside to cool.
5. In a large serving bowl, add arugula and basil. Add the roasted vegetables and gently toss. Add the cooked chicken and vinaigrette. Gently toss. Season with salt and pepper to taste. Let salad sit at room temperature for 20–30 minutes before serving.

FOOD EXCHANGES PER SERVING: 1½ VEGGIES, 1 GRAIN, 1 FAT

FIESTA SALMON (OR TURKEY!) BURGERS WITH A SIDE OF ARTICHOKE, SPINACH, AND TOMATO SALAD

Serves: 5

Burgers need not be a fat trap. Here, you can satisfy your burger craving with either omega-3-rich salmon or extra-lean ground turkey (do make sure it's extra lean though, as full-fat ground turkey can have practically the same amount of saturated fat content as beef!). You also want to make sure you purchase a healthy whole-grain bun, or better yet, try a *sprouted* whole-grain bun. Do note, this recipe makes five burgers, so you may have a little left over. The side of artichoke and tomato salad requires minimal hands-on time to prepare and it's just the thing to serve next to your yummy burger!

Fiesta Salmon (or Turkey!) Burgers:

1 pound wild salmon fillets (skin removed), cut into chunks, or 1 pound
    extra-lean ground turkey

½ of a red bell pepper, diced

2 teaspoons crushed garlic

3 tablespoons chopped cilantro

2 teaspoons Worcestershire sauce

2 scallions, whites and greens finely chopped

1 teaspoon cumin, divided

1 tablespoon *all-natural* taco seasoning (look for a brand without
    hydrogenated or partially hydrogenated oil)

¼ teaspoon salt, plus more to taste

Dash of cayenne

1 egg, lightly beaten (omega-3 organic egg, if possible)

⅓ cup whole-wheat panko crumbs (such as Ian's Natural Foods brand
available in supermarkets and at www.iansnaturalfoods.com)

2 fresh limes, halved

1 tablespoon canola oil mayonnaise (such as Hellmann's)

2 tablespoons all-natural BBQ sauce (look for a brand that does not use
    high-fructose corn syrup)

3 tablespoons prepared hummus (made with extra virgin olive oil, if
    possible)

5 sprouted whole-grain buns, toasted (such as Food for Life brand)

Note: You will also need parchment paper.

1. If using salmon, place chunks (uncooked) in a food processor. Pulse until you have ground salmon.
2. Place ground salmon or ground turkey in a large bowl. Add red bell pepper, garlic, cilantro, Worcestershire sauce, scallions, ½ teaspoon cumin, taco seasoning, salt, and a dash of cayenne. Mix ingredients well. Add egg and panko crumbs and mix thoroughly. Divide the mixture into five even portions and shape patties about 4 inches wide and ¾ inch thick. Season burgers lightly on both sides with salt. Transfer to a parchment-lined baking sheet and cover with plastic wrap. Refrigerate for 10–45 minutes.
3. Spray a large non-stick skillet with extra virgin olive oil cooking spray and heat over medium-high heat. Add burgers to hot skillet and cook 3–4 minutes per side, or until cooked through. Squeeze fresh lime juice on top of each burger.
4. In a small bowl, whisk together the canola oil, mayonnaise, BBQ sauce, hummus, and remaining ½ teaspoon cumin. Brush each burger with the sauce and serve at once on toasted buns.

FOOD EXCHANGES PER SERVING: 3 PROTEIN, 2½ GRAINS, 1 FAT

Artichoke, Spinach, and Tomato Salad:
2 packages (10 ounces each) frozen artichoke hearts
2 teaspoons extra virgin olive oil
Salt, to taste
¼ cup diced red onion
1 cup halved cherry tomatoes
2 teaspoons crushed garlic
1 tablespoon fresh lime juice
¼ cup chopped cilantro
1 tablespoon flaxseed oil (such as Barlean's)
Dash of cayenne pepper
3 cups baby spinach leaves

1. Preheat oven to 400 degrees.
2. Place frozen artichokes on a baking sheet. Drizzle with extra virgin olive oil and sprinkle with salt to taste. Roast artichokes for 40 minutes. Set aside to cool.

3. Place cooled artichokes in a medium-sized serving bowl. Add onion, tomatoes, garlic, lime juice, cilantro, and flaxseed oil. Gently toss. Season with salt and a dash of cayenne. Add the spinach. Toss again and serve.

FOOD EXCHANGES PER SERVING: 1 VEGGIE, 1 FAT

DESSERT

CREAMY MANGO-RASPBERRY FREEZE

Serves: 2

This decadent treat dishes waves of flavor with significantly fewer calories, less sugar, less saturated fat, and more nutrients than standard ice cream. It's the perfect dessert to share with your hubby after you put the munchkins to bed.

½ cup low-fat Greek style yogurt (such as Fage)
1 tablespoon sugar
¼ teaspoon pure lemon extract
½ cup frozen mango chunks
1 cup frozen raspberries
½ cup all-natural vanilla ice cream (such as Breyer's)

1. In a small bowl, mix together the yogurt, sugar, and lemon extract.
2. Put the yogurt mixture in a blender. Add the frozen mango and raspberries. Add the ice cream. Pulse several times until ingredients are well blended, but consistency is somewhat chunky. Serve at once.

FOOD EXCHANGES PER SERVING: 1 FRUIT, 1 GRAIN, ½ FAT

SPICED PUMPKIN CUSTARD WITH CARAMEL SAUCE

Serves: 8

Spanish-style flan was the inspiration for this nutrient-rich and decadent dessert. This version is actually more flavorful than traditional flan thanks to the spike of spice, and the addition of pumpkin packs additional flavor and a fiber punch too. It's also got a hefty dose of tofu (shhhh . . . mum's the word!).

10 ounces soft tofu (eyeball about ¾ package of a standard 14-ounce container of tofu, such as Nasoya brand)

1¼ cups sugar, divided

12 ounces low-fat evaporated milk

5 whole eggs plus 2 egg yolks (use omega-3 organic eggs, if possible)

¾ cup solid-pack canned pumpkin

1 teaspoon pure vanilla extract

1 teaspoon cinnamon

1 teaspoon ground ginger

¼ teaspoon ground nutmeg

¼ teaspoon salt

1. Preheat oven to 350 degrees. Put oven rack in middle position. Place a 2-quart soufflé dish or round ceramic casserole dish in the oven to warm while making caramel.

2. Remove tofu from package and wrap in paper towels or cheesecloth. Let sit 5–10 minutes to drain excess liquid.

3. Cook ¾ cup of the sugar in a very dry 2-quart heavy saucepan over moderate heat, undisturbed, until it begins to melt. Continue to cook, stirring occasionally with a fork, until sugar melts into a golden caramel. Carefully remove the soufflé dish from the oven, using mitts, and immediately pour the caramel into the dish, tilting the dish to evenly cover the bottom. Set dish aside and let caramel harden. Keep the oven on.

4. Place the drained tofu, milk, eggs, egg yolks, pumpkin, vanilla, cinnamon, ginger, nutmeg, and salt in a blender. Process 2 minutes, until very smooth and creamy. Add the remaining ¾ cup of sugar and blend until smooth and creamy. Pour the custard over the caramel in the dish.

5. Set soufflé dish in a water bath and cook custard for 1 hour and 25 minutes. Remove the dish from the water and transfer to a wire rack to cool. *(Note: Don't worry if custard is still a little runny when you remove it from the oven as it will firm up when chilled.)* Chill the custard in the refrigerator for at least 6 hours. To serve, carefully run a thin knife between the custard and the sides of the dish to loosen. Gently shake the dish until the custard jiggles. Invert a large platter with a lip over the dish. Holding the dish and platter securely, quickly invert and turn out custard onto a platter (caramel will pour over the top). Serve chilled.

FOOD EXCHANGES PER SERVING: 1 PROTEIN, 2½ GRAINS

HONEY-ROASTED PEACHES TOPPED WITH LEMONY CREAM

Serves: 1

Roasting fruit is one of the easiest ways to intensify and enhance its natural sweetness without adding globs of sugar. Here, the unexpected combination of sweet (from the fruit) and savory (from the lemony cream topping) makes a satisfyingly decadent treat that's surprisingly nutritious and light.

2 Georgia peaches, halved and pitted
4 teaspoons raw honey, divided
2 teaspoons lemon juice
¼ cup fat-free Greek-style plain yogurt (such as Fage)
2 tablespoons crème fraiche
½ teaspoon pure lemon extract

1. Preheat oven to 425 degrees. Spray a baking sheet with canola oil cooking spray. Place peaches cut side up on the baking sheet. Spread ½ teaspoon honey on each peach half. Drizzle lemon juice on top of peaches. Roast peaches for 25 minutes, or until soft. Remove peaches from oven, transfer to serving plates, and refrigerate until cold, about 30 minutes.

2. In a small bowl, whisk together the yogurt, crème fraiche, lemon extract, and remaining 2 teaspoons of honey. Spoon lemony cream on top of chilled peaches and serve.

FOOD EXCHANGES PER SERVING: ½ DAIRY, 2 FRUIT, 1 GRAIN, 1 FAT

GRILLED PINEAPPLE KABOBS WITH EASY FRUIT DIP

Serves: 2

Grilling fruit is the simplest, sweetest, and healthiest way to end a barbeque. You can grill just about any fruit you like, but pineapples are especially delicious. To make your treat extra special, just whip up the creamy easy fruit dip, and voila! Guiltless dessert in a flash.

¼ cup fat-free Greek-style yogurt (such as Fage)
¼ cup Neufatchel cream cheese
¼ cup low-fat ricotta
2 tablespoons lemon juice
1 tablespoon pure maple syrup
½ teaspoon pure almond extract
Extra virgin olive oil, for oiling grill rack
2½ cups pineapple chunks, cut into 1-inch squares
2 bamboo skewers, soaked in water for 30 minutes

1. In a small bowl, whisk together the yogurt, cream cheese, ricotta, lemon juice, maple syrup, and almond extract. Set aside.
2. Prepare a charcoal or gas grill for direct-heat grilling over medium-high heat. Oil the grill rack with extra virgin olive oil.
6. Thread pineapple chunks onto each skewer. Using tongs, place kabobs over the hottest part of the fire and grill, turning as needed, until lightly marked on each side, about 3 minutes total. Transfer kabobs to a serving plate and serve with dipping sauce.

FOOD EXCHANGES PER SERVING: ½ PROTEIN, 2½ FRUIT, ½ GRAIN, 1 FAT

Team Mallett Success Story

··

Courtney Scrabeck, 32, Altadena, CA

Lost

30 pounds

2 dress sizes

22 total inches

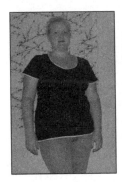 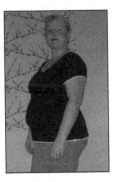

Before

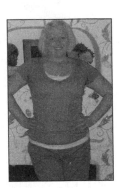

After

• • • ♦ ♦

Before going on the Super Fit Mama program, Courtney weighed 200 pounds. "I had two kids in two years and after all that my body didn't feel like it belonged to me, but to my babies," she says. "I desperately wanted to feel like me again instead of an enormous breastfeeding cow." Though Courtney wanted to lose at least 40 pounds, her goals were bigger than that. "I wanted to be healthy," she adds. "I couldn't sleep at night and was exhausted all the time."

Her favorite part of the program was the meal plan and the simple way it explains portion sizes. "I think anyone can learn to eat better with this plan," she says. Before, Courtney was eating large portions of whatever she wanted, which was mostly junk food. But once she started the plan, she realized how full she could get on a lot less food, especially when she traded processed, high-fat, high-calorie edibles for healthy options like protein and lots and lots of vegetables, which she says were "no guilt." The plan also taught her about balance and eating in the real world, not dieting. "I knew that if I had a piece of bacon with breakfast, I wouldn't eat a chicken sandwich for lunch."

Even more amazing than getting her eating under control was the fact that Courtney went from never exercising to eagerly looking forward to breaking a sweat at least five times a week. "I loved how the workouts were divided into short increments," she says. "I always thought that Pilates was only for super fit dancer types, but I felt better about my midsection after only a week of the Super Fit Mama Pilates-inspired moves." Now, Courtney's confidence is through the roof. "I feel better about myself and less 'Mom' like," she says. "I can wear clothes from regular stores, sleep like a rock, have more energy, and stand up straighter, and I'm so much more motivated to eat right and exercise than I was before."

MOTIVATION FROM
TEAM MALLETT

"Before the Super Fit Mama program, my family and I ate lots of drive-thru because it was quick. But the food plan and recipes are so easy too and make me realize that all it takes is a little planning and thinking ahead to eat right. I love that I am setting a good example for my family with both the working out *and* eating right."
—Erica Shepherd

"A good little tidbit that I heard a long time ago is this quote: 'Nothing tastes as good as losing weight feels.' Isn't that the truth!!!!"
—Tara Kali

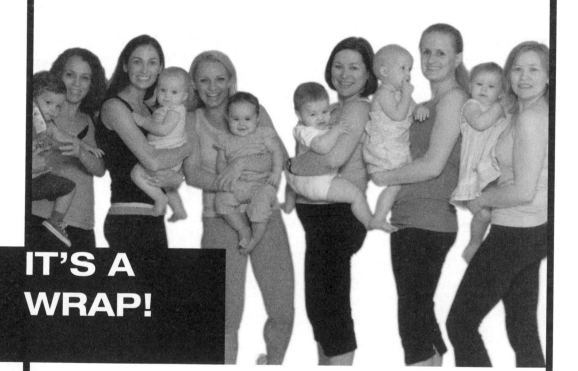

CHAPTER 12

IT'S A
WRAP!

REMEMBER THE LAST WEEK OF MY FIRST PREGNANCY, I JUST couldn't believe that I was almost at my due date—that due date that ran through my mind daily for nine months. That due date that was circled in red on my calendar. I couldn't believe that when people asked me how far along I was, I could tell them my baby was "Due this week." (Which of course made them step back since they feared I'd deliver the baby right then and there.) I couldn't believe that soon enough my pregnancy would be over. Well, that's how I feel about being at the end of this book. I can't believe it's done—and if you started the Super Fit Mama plan when you were pregnant and stuck with it while your baby came into the world and reached several important developmental milestones, I'm sure you're wondering where the time has gone, too. By now, you have reached some important milestones of your own. I'm willing to bet you feel more comfortable in your own skin and actually like what you see when you catch a glimpse of yourself in the mirror.

There's a new spring in your step, because no matter where you are on your journey to a fitter, healthier you, the fact that you're taking action to feel your best is something to be proud of. It's so empowering to feel good about yourself and to realize that you are important and worth the effort.

Naturally, just because the book (and your official postpartum period) is over doesn't mean that your road to wellness has come to an end, too. In fact, it's only just begun. Being a Super Fit Mama is not just for a few months: All the tools you have learned through this program are lifestyle changes that you can carry with you forever. Sure, there will be setbacks along the way, and there will be times when things feel overwhelming, but that is life. It's normal. It's human nature. This does not mean that you have failed or that you will never achieve your goal; it just means that you will need to take a little detour and get ready to go again.

And you now have the experience you will need to navigate yourself back to the path that leads to success. Life and motherhood are two things that are very unpredictable (to say the least!), and we just have to go with the flow and set realistic expectations for ourselves. Though I aim to exercise every day, there are those times when I just can't fit it in (and unless someone could magically make my day twenty-five hours long instead of twenty-four whenever I asked, it will continue to be like that from time to time). I am disappointed when this happens, but I don't let it ruin my good intentions. I move on and accept that it's going to happen. I don't let it affect my mood; I just remind myself that this is the best I can do right now and try to make up for it the next time.

You also have to remember that every healthy step you take is making your family healthier, too. They notice when mom slips on her workout clothes and will follow your healthy lead and exercise, too. I remember once when my daughter was about four years old and I was with her at a playdate. The other mom mentioned how she never exercised and I guess Amber overheard her. When we left their house, Amber looked at me with huge eyes and whispered, "Mom, Julie's mom doesn't exercise!" Her tone was about what it would have been if she was saying that Julie's mom didn't brush her teeth or shower. At first I found it strange, but then I realized that my daughter saw exercise as a natural part of daily life and that she didn't know otherwise. You can teach the same lesson with healthy eating. I don't know how many times I've said this in the book, but what you eat, your family eats, and this starts when they're in vitro. You set the standards now and always. If you've never before in your life been inspired to eat clean, the time is now.

Do you remember when you were young and you thought you were just so invincible? I loved that feeling because it seemed like nothing could ever touch me. However, after decades of living and after having children you realize that you're not so invincible, and that's a scary thought when your family is the most important thing in your life. I want to make sure that I can prevent illnesses for myself and my family, something that good nutritious foods and regular exercise have been proven to do.

The wonderful women of Team Mallett are now living in their pre-pregnancy bodies and pre-pregnancy wardrobes, and some say they look better than before their pregnancy (and their husbands aren't disputing that!). However, what so many of them told me is that, though they started this program focused only on fitting into their favorite jeans again, they now view it as so much more. They feel healthier and sexier and want to maintain that feeling. They have learned that Super Fit Mama isn't just something you do for nine months or even twenty months, but something you can do for life.

Enjoy the journey of motherhood. It's the experience of a lifetime, and the only downside is that it goes way too quickly. My life would not be complete without my two beautiful children; through them I've been able to find the true me. I love the old saying that "practice makes perfect," but in this case it should be "practice makes progress." I hope I have helped you kick-start your life as an active, healthy mother, and I urge you to keep up the good work. I wish you all the luck in the world.

And never forget: You deserve to be a Super Fit Mama!

Cover photo is Katherine Findley Smiley, who was ten months, as you will agree the perfect cover model.

The mom-to-be model in Chapter 2, "First Trimester Fitness," is Lori Montgomery, a physical therapist and now a proud mom for the first time, of Joshua.

The mom-to-be model in Chapter 4, "Third Trimester Fitness," is Rory Olivarez, a Pilates Professional and now a mom of three with her new addition to the family, Lucia Elena Olivarez.

The photos in "Baby Workouts On the Go," Chapter 8, are of Coco Serrio, who was all of eight weeks, Angelina Joy Benton, who was nine months old, and Kieran Jeffcoat, who was 13 months old.

FITNESS EQUIPMENT

For all your fitness products (weights, mats, and bands), go to:
www.optp.com
www.spriproducts.com
www.fitnesswholesale.com
www.target.com
www.fleurville.com (for the Zafu bolsters featured in the Pregnancy
section)

EXERCISE DVDS

My DVDs are available for purchase in retail stores and online. The following are websites where you can purchase a variety of videos:
www.traceymallett.com
www.amazon.com
www.collage.com

RUNNING STROLLERS

Go to www.Babyjogger.com for running strollers like the ones featured
in this book.

YUMMY HEALTHY FOODS AND DRINKS

As you know, eating healthy is important to me. Here are some of my favorite companies and products. Check them out. I know you won't be disappointed.

Amy's Kitchen soups and other products: www.amyskitchen.com

Barlean's flaxseeds and flaxseed oil: www.barleans.com

BellyBar: www.nuribella.com

Biochem Whey Protein: www.biochem-fitness.com/pages/powders_main.html

Dannon Activia Yogurt: www.dannon.com

Drink Hint: www.drinkhint.com

Fage yogurts: www.fageusa.com

Food for Life whole-grain sprouted breads, pastas, and tortilla: www.foodforlife.com

Ghirardelli baking chocolate: www.ghirardelli.com

Hellmann's mayonnaise: www.hellmanns.com

Ian's products: www.iansnaturalfoods.com

King Arthur flours and baking mixes: www.kingarthurflour.com

Lara Bars: www.larabar.com

Muir Glen Organic tomato products and sauces: www.muirglen.com

Nasoya tofu: www.nasoya.com

Nature's Path cereals and breads: www.naturespath.com

Organic Valley dairy products and omega-3 eggs: www.organicvalley.coop

Pacific Natural Foods: www.pacificfoods.com

Quaker Oats: www.quakeroats.com

Really Raw Honey: www.reallyrawhoney.com

Silk soy milk products: www.silksoymilk.com

Stonyfield Farm yogurt: www.stonyfield.com

Toufayan Pita: www.toufayan.com

Vitalicious VitaMuffin: www.vitalicious.com

Weider products: www.weider.com

MOMMY PRODUCTS

I love the beauty products from Mama Mio. To get a FREE 30-milliliter Boob Tube bust-firming cream with any Mama Mio order at www.mamamio.com, enter **SUPERFIT** at checkout. Limit one per customer. Cannot be combined with any other offer.

CLOTHING

These are some of my favorite sources of stylish clothes for working out or just for hanging out and looking hot!

www.hardtailforever.com

www.rogiani.com

www.fitmaternity.com (great selection of maternity fitness clothes)

www.destinationmaternity.com

SHOES

I love Earth Footwear because every pair of shoes incorporates "Negative Heel Technology." That means your toes are 3.7 degrees higher than your heels, which helps to realign your body and promotes good posture. See www.earth.us.

For running and impact activities, I like Asics shoes because they give great arch and foot support. See www.asics.com.

INFORMATION WEB SITES

Here are some Web sites offering valuable information on health and wellness:

Aerobics and Fitness Association of America: www.afaa.com

American Academy on Exercise: www.ace.com

American Journal of Clinical Nutrition: www.ajcn.org/cgi/content/full/69/5/959

BabyCenter: www.babycenter.com

Ban Trans Fat Information Site: www.bantransfat.com

TheBump: www.thebump.com

Centers for Disease Control and Prevention: www.cdc.gov

Child Birth Connection: www.childbirthconnection.org

Consumer Reports: www.consumerreports.org/healthaccess

The Federal Government Source for Women's Health: www.4woman
.gov/pregnancy

Food pyramid: www.mypyramid.gov

Medline Plus: www.nlm.nih.gov/medlineplus/pregnancy.html

National Agricultural Library (SDA Nutrient Database): www.nal.us da
.gov

WebMD: www.webmd.com

DOWNLOADABLE WORKOUTS

Go to www.iamplify.com to download my audio workouts.

You can download any of my videos to your computer, cell phone, or mp3 player at www.mypypeline.com.

VIDEO ON DEMAND

Check your local cable listing for Exercise TV, where you can find hundreds of workouts to choose from, including mine. See www.exercisetv.tv.

FOOD LOG

	Protein	Dairy	Grains	Fruits	Fats	Veggies (nonstarches)	Water
Breakfast	P P P P	D D	G G	F	FATS	V V V	W W
Snack	P P	D D	G	F F		V V V	W
Lunch	P P P P	D D	G G	F	FATS	V V V	W W
Snack	P P	D D	G	F F		V V V	W
Dinner	P P P P	D D	G G	F	FATS	V V V	W W
Evening snack (optional)	P P	D D	G	F F	FATS	V V V	W
Day's Maximum						Unlimited	Unlimited

DAY'S TOTAL

Journal Your Treat:

Daily Notes:

WORKOUT LOG

	MON	TUES	WED	THUR	FRI	SAT	SUN
A.M.							DAY OFF
LUNCH							
P.M.							
TOTAL FITNESS SEGMENTS							
BONUS CARDIO							
COMMENTS							

Progress Sheet

Fill out the sheet every 2 weeks   Dates/Week # _____ to _____

Beginning Weight: _____   End Weight: _____

How do your clothes feel?

Beginning   *End*

Loose? _____   Tight: _____   Looser? _____   No change: _____

MEASUREMENTS

WAIST

Beginning: _____   End: _____

HIPS

Beginning: _____   End: _____

THIGHS

Beginning   End

Right: _____   Left: _____   Right: _____   Left: _____

CHEST

Beginning: _____   End: _____

ARMS (in between shoulder & elbow)

Beginning   End

Right: _____   Left: _____   Right: _____   Left: _____

Energy levels

Beginning: _____   End: _____

How do you feel overall?

Beginning: _____   End: _____

A special thanks to the following people for their generous contributions to this book.

WENDY CRUMP, RD

Wendy Crump is a registered dietitian and founder of Kids on the Run. She has dedicated the past fifteen years to teaching and empowering families to live healthier lives. She holds a bachelor's degree in dietetics from the University of California, Davis, and is the author of "Healthy Families for Life" on The Capessa Blog: Sharing the Wisdom of Women on Yahoo! Health. For more information, visit www.kids-on-the-run.com.

DALE ALLEYNE-HO, HON., E.C.E., CCBE, LE

Dale Alleyne-Ho has been guiding expectant couples throughout the process of pregnancy, childbirth, and beyond for over six years as a Certified Childbirth/Lactation Educator and Early Childhood/Parent Educator. She is also founder of Learning for Life (www.learning4lyf.ca) and the proud mom of four.

LAURA HORN, MPT

Laura Horn is a mother of two and a physical therapist specializing in women's health at ATP Physical Therapy in South Pasadena, California. She is a member of a multidisciplinary team at University of Southern

California University Hospital, which coordinates the delivery of care to patients with pelvic floor dysfunction, and a part-time faculty member at Mount St. Mary's College in the Doctorate of Physical Therapy Program. She is also involved in research on the topics of Pilates and women's health.

HEATHER JEFFCOAT, DPT

Heather Jeffcoat is a physical therapist, writer, and educator with a quarterly column in the International Childbirth Education Association Journal entitled "Perinatal Wellness."

She also teaches wellness and restorative classes around the Greater Los Angeles area and continues to treat patients with Women's Health and general orthopedic diagnoses. See *www.thepilatespt.com*.

HOWARD S. KAUFMAN, MD, MBA

Howard S. Kaufman is associate professor of clinical surgery and vice chairman for patient safety and quality in the Department of Surgery at the Keck School of Medicine at the University of Southern California. His primary clinical and research interests and expertise are in multimodality treatment of colorectal cancer, the multidisciplinary treatment of pelvic floor disorders, and the correlations between obesity and colon cancer and obesity and pelvic floor dysfunction.

Before relocating to Southern California, he was the codirector of the multidisciplinary Pelvic Floor Disorders Program at the Johns Hopkins Hospital in Baltimore, Maryland. In 2002, Dr. Kaufman established the Center of Pelvic Floor Disorders at the University of Southern California, and he continues to direct this multidisciplinary center, which attracts patients from all over the United States. He is a member of numerous medical and surgical societies, has coauthored sixty peer-reviewed manuscripts and fifteen book chapters, and directs an active research program currently engaged in more than fifteen clinical and translational investigations. Last year he was honored as a "Top Doctor" in the San Gabriel Valley in the specialty of colon and rectal surgery by Pasadena magazine.

Dr. Kaufman is in the process of relocating his programs in colorectal and pelvic floor disorders to be primarily affiliated with the Huntington Hospital in Pasadena, California.

IVY LARSON, ACSM

Ivy Larson is a healthy lifestyle coach and ACSM certified health fitness instructor. Along with her husband, Andrew Larson, MD, she authored The Whole Foods Diet Cookbook, The Gold Coast Cure, and The Gold Coast Cure's Fitter, Firmer, Faster Program. She lives with her family in North Palm Beach, Florida, where she conducts "Health and Body Lifestyle Makeover Programs" as well as whole foods cooking classes at Whole Foods Market. See www.the2Larsons.com.

MERRILL SUE LEWEN, MD

Merrill Sue Lewen is a gynecologist who is currently in practice in Houston, Texas, with Town and Country Gynecology in the Memorial area. Her particular interest now is menopausal medicine and adolescent gynecology, although her practice is a general one. Dr. Lewen has two young teenagers, and it was during her pregnancies with them that her interest in exercise and pregnancy began. Currently she either swims, runs, or does yoga every day. Her approach to patients is holistic and includes emphasis on a well-balanced diet, exercise, meaningful relationships, and having fun.

ACKNOWLEDGMENTS

Wow, I can't believe I'm finally sitting here right now writing the last piece of this long awaited book. My personal journey with *Super Fit Mama* has had so many loops and turns, I really had many doubts that this book would ever come to fruition. Yet, I am so proud to say it's done and excited to share with the world. However, there are so many people I have to thank, without them my dream would have never came true.

First, I'd like to thank my fabulous literary agent Linda Konner for finding me a home with Da Capo Press not just for this book but also for *Sexy in 6*. Next, is Michele Bender who truly has a way with words, thanks for always giving me your honest opinion.

Then, I'd also like to give a big hug to all the people who contributed to my book, especially Merrell Lewin, Howard Kaufman, Laura Horn, and Wendy Crump. Last but not least the beautiful models that spent many hours posing for the pictures and Team Mallett who are my inspiration for never giving up and allowing their dreams to come true. Thanks guys for making this book relatable to all you women out there striving for a healthier lifestyle.

Super Fit Mama is for my family who are my rock and my children who are my life. I love you all so much; we really are the **Super Fit Family!!**

The Total Body Mommy Makeover System

If you loved this book, you will love the accompanying DVDs too! Work out with Tracey Mallett directly from your living room and put the Super Fit Mama plan into action on a daily basis.

Exercise safely through pregnancy and finally get your body back after baby!

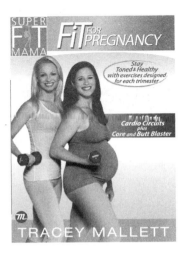
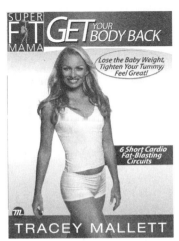
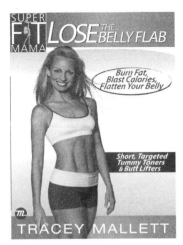

Join Team Mallett at www.teammallett.com where you can make friends and get support from other women.

To purchase, visit www.traceymallett.com
or www.amazon.com

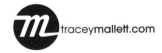
traceymallett.com